EFT Tapping - Learn in 5 Min

The Effective Tapping Solution

for
Anxiety, Addictions, Weight Loss & Wealth

by Using
the Tapping Therapy

PRAISE FOR
"EFT Tapping - Learn in 5 Min."

"Right from the start, the book jumps right into the information in a very straightforward and easy to understand style. Buckland uses a lot of simple analogies that really drive home his points and it's presented in a way that forgoes fluff for easy to understand concepts and step-by-step methods. It's a great way for beginners to start utilizing the tapping technique in their daily lives.

Though I can't personally speak for physical illnesses, I noticed a significant improvement in stress, anxiety, and general emotional wellbeing when using the techniques listed in the book. It seems odd at first, but the principles presented in this book are quite similar to (and even draw from) well-founded practices such as acupressure, self-affirmation, and holism (the practice of healing the whole body, rather than focusing on one aspect or symptom alone).

Whether you intend to utilize these techniques in your own life, or are simply studying the methods of holistic wellness, this book is certainly an interesting read." - *Samuel Reese*

"As a Psychologist, I have been working within the fields of psychotherapy for over 17 years. During that time I treated many treatments seeking to effectively reduce anxiety and panic attacks. After reading Buckland's book and after I have applied the "EFT Tapping - Learn in 5 Min: The Effective Tapping Solution for Anxiety, Addictions, Weight Loss & Wealth by Using the Tapping Therapy" - I must say: none of my classic treatments come close to the Tapping Therapy. Buckland himself as a clinical therapist understands the nature of anxiety and panic disorders and its success to explain it on his book is not just a theoretical concepts as well as a plain and easy EFT techniques that, when applied, provide the complete cure for stress and anxiety. The EFT Tapping - Learn in 5 min is highest recommend it to anyone suffering from stress, anxiety and panic attacks." - *Dr. A. Robbins*

"I am a licensed therapist TFT (Thought Field Therapy) and I know therefore that tapping therapy is effective. This book is well written and instructions are easy to follow. Recommend this book to everyone." - *Terje Myrvang*

"The author does an awesome job on explaining EFT, its benefits and how easy it is to learn. The best part about EFT is you can do it yourself and it's free! Relieving stress, anxiety, depression, obesity, etc. without using drugs or needles (acupuncture) is always a big plus. The author not only gives you the techniques for tapping he also prepares you for the therapy. It is also great to know that this method does not have any side effects." - *Alicia Ellison Grant*

"This book doesn't waste your time, it is right to the point and effectively shares the basic EFT techniques you can put into practice today to manage your physical or emotional illness. Also, I believe his background in NLP has helped him share the instructions in such a way that is easy to follow, internalize, and remember.

If, like me, you are just getting introduced to EFT through this book then you will find it very informing. Can't talk about those who already know it though as I am quite new to the technique n happy to have learned about it through Buckland's book." – *Zara*

"This is the second book I've read on the subject of tapping pressure points for de-stressing. In the first book, it was just a part of a larger book. This book is completely devoted to the subject of Emotional Tapping Therapy. Naturally, as I read it, I had to tap the suggested spots on the body. It was amazing how quickly I felt better!" - *Java Davis*

"A year ago my anxiety was so strong. Since I learned EFT by reading your EFT Tapping book, anytime I leave the house, I feel a fearless sense of mastery of any social situation. Before EFT I felt a lot of anxiety about the future. I was restless and didn't sleep well. Since starting EFT I'm calmer and don't concern myself as much with what is going to happen tomorrow." **-** *Dian Austin*

"I have been suffering with my anxiety for the last few years and I feel it's getting worse. I started thinking nobody could help me and I would have to live with this for the rest of my life. Then I found "EFT Tapping - Learn in 5 Min". When I first started reading the content and listening to what Ben Buckland had to say about EFT Tapping to overcome anxiety, I instantly knew this was someone who understands what I was going through and can help me. Tapping every day gives me so much reassurance and confidence to start putting things in place to begin my road to recovery. I have never looked back since!" - *Daniel Silva*

"This book is an excellent guide and introduction to EFT tapping on how it can help heal one's problems and illnesses. The clear defined plan and instructions within the book on how one should approach and adopt the "recipe" on using the EFT tapping method, are very easy to follow and understand.

The author also does a fantastic job at explaining in detail about each of the steps involved, how to prepare you properly beforehand, as well as providing daily-life relatable examples to help one understand the topic better. Overall a great and useful book you can get started right away." - *Sky Nealon*

ABOUT THE AUTHOR

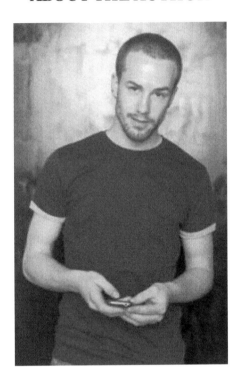

Ben Buckland was always attracted to eastern philosophy. It was this interest that drew him to the teachings and practices of The Tapping Therapy (EFT). He studied Chinese medicine, Qigong and **Advanced EFT Practitioner, EFT Certified Trainer and Master NLP Practitioner.**

Buckland writes his books to give you clear insights and identify your positive point of view and reveal your blind spots, and his EFT TAPPING book help you and implement your path toward the life you've always dreamed of.

Buckland studied Positive Psychology with a special interest in health psychology and the interaction of the mind and body. Over the past years, he has worked with anxiety disorder patients. He run workshops on coping with stress and anxiety, binge eating, and much more. His work experience includes individual EFT Tapping Therapy, Behavioral Psychology, and personal training.

Blog: eft-tapping-therapy.blogspot.com

Facebook: facebook.com/eft.tapping.therapy.solution

Twitter: @kdpbenbuckland

Email: kdpbuckland@gmail.com

Table of Contents

Introduction   **2**

Part 1: Tapping for Stress, Anxiety and Emotional Problems

Chapter 1: What is EFT?   **7**

Chapter 2: EFT Research   **14**

Chapter 3: The Body's Energy System and the Tapping Points   **18**

Chapter 4: The Four Steps of Basic EFT Application   **26**

Part 2: Get Your Food Control Back Tapping for Weight Loss

Chapter 5: Weight loss and the Reality of Emotions   **43**

Chapter 6: The Basic Recipe for Weight Loss   **50**

Chapter 7: Taming Hunger Pangs   **59**

Chapter 8: Optimizing Your Metabolism with EFT   **67**

Chapter 9: Addressing Self-Acceptance with EFT   **79**

Part 3: Tapping for Wealth Tapping for Financial Abundance

Chapter 10: Money and your Internal Beliefs about Wealth and Financial Abundance   **83**

Chapter 11: Reasons why the Law of Attraction isn't working for you   **86**

Chapter 12: How can EFT raise your Vibration?   **89**

Chapter 13: The Basic Recipe for Attracting Money and Financial Wealth   **95**

Chapter 14: Advanced EFT Tapping Scripts - Cleaning Negative Beliefs about Money   **105**

Chapter 15: Advanced EFT Tapping Scripts - Producing your Positive "Wealth Frequency" that Transforms your Relationships to Money   114

Chapter 16: Advanced EFT Tapping Scripts - Manifesting and Attracting Wealth and Financial Abundance   121

Part 4: Tapping for Improving Relationships

Chapter 17: Improving Relationships   131

Part 5: Tapping for Other Common Issues

Chapter 18: Tapping for Kids   151

Chapter 19: Tapping for Enhancing Sports Performance   156

Chapter 20: Tapping for Sleep Problems   159

Chapter 21: Tapping for Self Confidence   161

Part 6: The Stress Release Tapping Challenge - BONUS   182

Conclusion   250

PUBLISHER'S DISCLAIMER

The material in this book is for informational purposes only. As each individual situation is unique, you should use proper discretion, in consultation with a health care practitioner, before undertaking the exercises and techniques described in this book. If you have any health problems, consult a Doctor before using this book. The author and publisher expressly disclaim responsibility for any adverse effects that may result from the use or application of the book.

Introduction

EFT Tapping - Emotional Freedom Technique - is a fast evolving treatment and is often referred to as "Psychological acupressure". The Tapping technique works by releasing energy blockages within the energy system which are the source of emotional problems. The Tapping Therapy uses the natural healing abilities of the mind and body, providing opportunities to achieving physical and emotional well-being in a faster time.

The Tapping Therapy is based on the concept that memories, beliefs, and negative emotions are stored in the body as energy. These emotions and beliefs can cause problems such as eating disorders, phobias, low self-esteem, depression, and addiction.

This book contains plain and easy steps on how to overcome phobias, anxieties, addictions, food cravings and other emotional problems – by using the powerful practice of Eft Tapping. It is very simple, and can be used effectively as a self-help tool, which empowers people to actively contribute to their own healing and development process.

You will learn concepts and ideas on how you can use EFT for weight loss. Oftentimes, people who want to shed pounds focus too much on dieting and forget to deal with the real issues that have pushed them to become overweight.
The book will help you understand what habits and traits lead to emotional eating and suggest tapping strategies that help you reprogram your outlook towards food and yourself.

In addition, you will learn proven steps and strategies on how to effectively apply and practice EFT tapping therapy to be able to attract wealth and financial abundance and in a way improve one's quality of life and change one's negative beliefs and behavior to positive outlook and attitude.

Many people believe that we attract what we think about. This is precisely what the law of attraction is all about and this eBook will seek to provide the significant relationship between the law of attraction and EFT tapping therapy. You will know the reasons why the law of attraction seems not to be working for you and what you can do to change your mindset into positive energy to attract success and financial abundance.

With The Tapping Therapy, health, wealth and happiness are at YOUR fingertips!

How to use this book?
I have tried to make this book easy to use. If you wish to learn tapping in 5 min - please pay attention to this $\sqrt{}$ sign. This sign means - it is a must read and very important part to follow.

I hope you enjoy it!

Thank You,
Ben Buckland

Part 1
Tapping Therapy – The Concepts

Tapping for Stress, Anxiety
and Emotional Problems

Chapter 1: What is EFT?

Back to Basics

When things get too complicated, the best way to recover is to go back to basics. This trend is easy to spot in fashion. Remember the little black dress that never goes out of style? Or the basic white tee that goes well with a funky scarf? In any event, wearing these pieces still make you fashionable whatever the season.

Similarly, natural healing methods are making a comeback in the field of medicine. As conspiracy theories between pharmaceutical companies and health professionals proliferate; and the cost of treatments continues to rise, more and more people are turning to natural healing techniques that are less invasive yet effective. Among these methods, Emotional Freedom Techniques, also known as EFT or EFT Tapping, emerged as a new field that deals with emotional issues to promote faster physical recovery.

Defining EFT

EFT is a healing technique that works on this basic premise: *"The disruption of the body's energy system is the primary cause of any negative emotion."* Any kind of emotional stress disrupts the natural flow of energy in the body. As a result, the capacity of the body to heal itself is reduced.

Emotional Freedom Techniques or EFT which is also known as EFT tapping is a healing tool universally recognized to be able to provide remarkable outcome for emotional, performance and physical issues. The principle behind EFT lies in the belief that every aspect of human life that needs improvement carries in itself some unresolved issues of the emotions along the way. EFT also considers physical pain and discomfort or any other medical conditions to be connected and influenced by our emotional state and stress which can obstruct the flow of healing energy and potential inside our body.

Five thousand years ago, ancient Chinese physicians have discovered that energy, courses through the body via a complex network of energy circuits. These energy circuits became known as the meridians. The Chinese believed that the secret to a healthy body is the continuous flow of energy through these meridians. The problem is, sometimes the meridians get blocked and the energy accumulates in one point much like when water gets stuck behind a dam wall. A disruption in the natural energy flow within the body limits its capability to heal itself, leading to the development of illnesses.

EFT is a healing tool that declogs blocked energy circuits in two steps:

Step 1:
Letting a patient mentally tune into a specific self-issue;

Step 2:
Stimulation of the meridian points throughout the body by tapping on them with the fingertips.

How does EFT tapping work?

The tapping motion in combination with the act of acknowledging a particular issue leads to the release of blockages in the energy system. As a result, the normal flow of energy in the body is restored, and the person feels better and becomes physically well after the treatment. The healing process is not instantaneous in some cases. More complex diseases may require more sessions of EFT to be fully well.

EFT is somehow related but not entirely similar to the acupuncture therapy. It mixes ancient wisdom of acupuncture and traditional talk therapy in the absence of needles. Instead of using needles to activate some energy points in the body, most of these acupuncture points can be stimulated just by tapping with one's fingertips while counseling or talk therapy is taking place simultaneously.

If other treatments and therapy aim to change how we view and think about something, EFT aims to change the way we feel about it. Usually, changing how we feel about some things lasts longer and is more effective and powerful when it comes to changing and influencing our way of life.

It was already observed and accepted by science and medical experts performing and reading functional MRI that stimulating some points on the layers of the skin does not only cause brain activities to change but it also deactivates the areas of the brain that activates whenever we experience fear and pain. Similarly, with stimulation of the acupuncture points through EFT tapping, the electrochemical level and electromagnetic level (which are both responsible for human emotion and feelings) also change significantly. This is what EFT tapping is all about.

The Origins of EFT

EFT stands for "Emotional Freedom Technique" and it was developed by Gary Craig. He said that EFT was created based on breakthroughs that gave many people a break from pain, illnesses, and emotional problems. EFT can be thought of as similar to acupuncture – except for the fact that instead of using needles, the energy meridian points in the body are stimulated by tapping them with the tips of the fingers. The process of executing EFT is quite easy to commit to memory and could be done wherever you may be.

The emotional freedom technique is founded on the concept that "the cause of all negative emotions is a disruption in the body's energy system, and our unresolved negative emotions are major contributors to most physical pains and diseases". EFT also obtains its powerful effect both from the traditional discoveries of the East (that have been employed as healing techniques for more than five thousand years) and from Albert Einstein's research (one of the greatest scientist of all time, proving that everything that exists in this world, including the human body, is made up of energy).

Western healing experts (aka the ones who represent mainstream medicine) have actually overlooked these two concepts and this is the reason why EFT frequently works where people in the Western world have failed (despite the use of powerful drugs). To put it simply, standard Western healing techniques have disregarded what was obvious all along.

The Benefits of EFT

Many people have already discovered that practicing EFT is not only very helpful in healing their physical illnesses and emotional issues, but it is also very valuable in calming down the voices inside their heads that tell them that they are not good enough or worthy of love, happiness, and success. EFT involves several techniques that allow people to use it for various applications. However, if you are just starting to learn EFT, it is ideal that you begin by studying the basic "recipe". As you become more confident in your EFT skills, you could then explore how you can be more creative in applying EFT in your life.

A lot of people ask the question: "Is EFT effective against *<insert whatever specific physical illness or emotional problem that they're currently facing>*?" Well, the answer to that question is both "yes" and "no".

Over the years, EFT has been very valuable in healing various kinds of physical illnesses including joint pains, headache, wart, nasal congestion, upset stomach, and even inflamed kidney. Similarly, there are a lot of people who reported that their emotional problems such as anger, loneliness, anxiety, mental block, lack of concentration, and sense of loss were eased because of applying emotional freedom techniques. There are even those who claim that EFT is effective in treating certain serious mental disorders, such as learning disabilities and autism. EFT was also successful in controlling excessive desire

11

for sweet and carbohydrate-rich foods. A lot of people have also quit smoking by applying the techniques of EFT. Because of all these success stories, we are led to believe that EFT could really prove to be valuable in a lot of areas that we may be working on. Gary Craig suggests that we could try EFT on everything, mainly because practicing EFT does not really have any negative side effect. All you really need to do is allot some time to do the actual tapping exercises.

Nonetheless, you need to keep two very critical things in your mind. First is that EFT works quickly on certain illnesses or problems, but it may require more time and effort in treating others. When you start practicing EFT, you will experience "one minute miracles", wherein you achieve complete relief even after just one round of tapping exercise. However, do not expect that you will have the same experience every time you perform tapping exercises. If you're finding that a bit difficult to understand, consider this simple fact – healing a torn muscle requires more time and more effort compared to healing a minor cut in your finger.

EFT works the same way – more serious illnesses will require more time and effort compared to minor ones. It is therefore very important that you keep realistic expectations when performing emotional freedom techniques.

The second thing that you need to know is that certain illnesses or problems are a lot more complex than others. Certain illnesses will definitely be very simple to resolve. Other illnesses or problems though, specifically those that took several years to develop, would be quite difficult to deal with. It is understandable that as a newbie, you might feel overwhelmed when you do not know at which specific point to start – and that is quite fine. All seasoned EFT practitioners all started as newbies once. You just need to be very patient with yourself, especially when it comes to progress. Do not easily give up when you cannot see any positive effects right away.

A lack of noticeable results simply implies that the EFT application that you are currently doing is not as effective as it should be. One good reason could be that you do not have the right EFT approach for the illness or problem that you are dealing with.

Chapter 2: EFT Research

Emotional Freedom Techniques are grouped under Energy Psychology since it involves the manipulation of energy within the body's meridians. As with other EP curative methods, EFT has been extensively studied for its effectiveness, especially because bioenergetic manipulation is new to Western science. So far, hundreds of EFT experiments were done and the results were published in credible scientific journals.

Numerous studies demonstrated that EFT has a high degree of possible effectiveness for treating certain physical and psychological complaints. Some of these are:

Depression. EFT was proven to relieve depression among different groups of people such as teenagers, psychology students, fibromyalgia and psoriasis patients, war veterans, PTSD sufferers, healthcare workers, and disaster survivors. A portion of these studies also point out that EFT goes beyond reducing sadness, but also affects the way distressing memories are mentally processed. An EFT session tames traumas so they don't cause powerful emotions when recalled after therapy.

Anxiety and phobias. There were experiments where EFT was used to treat various kinds of phobias, including fear of various animals, objects, scenarios and activities such as public speaking, test taking, and dental treatments. EFT was discovered to reduce anxiety levels even after a single session. Some critics point out that EFT is very similar to alternative methods used in one experiment, namely touching non-meridian arm locations and doll acupressure parts. This only shows that EFT is indeed effective, and even though other methods may do the same thing as EFT, it still produces the desired results. In fact, the group that didn't use the tapping techniques retained their phobias, which proves the efficacy of EFT tapping methods.

Pain. EFT was tested to determine whether it can provide relief to headache sufferrs, chronic illness patients, and stressed out individuals. The results show that EFT helps these people manage their pain by reducing both emotional distress and the actual physical sensations.

Addictions. Those who have intense cravings have found greater self control after using EFT methods. Weight watchers also benefitted from EFT because of its appetite-reducing effects.

Physical and Psychological Conditions. A study within the National Health Service in Sandwell, West Midlands involves treating people with varying physical and emotional complaints. Although there were only 31 people who finished the therapy, 30 of them showed remarkable results – a success rate of almost 100%. Aside from treating disorders effectively, EFT was seen to enhance abilities in sports and in school.

These well-documented reports signify that EFT is an effective treatment for a wide range of concerns. Although EFT is not thoroughly understood because it has non-scientific components, many researchers agree that EFT delivers what it promises.

Science Catching Up with EFT

EFT is based on an ancient Chinese system of knowledge combined with modern psychological research. Some of the less understood ideas behind EFT are the following:

Chi. The principles behind EFT involve subtle energy, which is largely unmeasured and unacknowledged by science. However, scientific breakthroughs hint at the presence of these invisible forces that mystics and psychics have known for millenia. For example, Kirlian photography makes it possible to capture the energetic field surrounding and interpenetrating living beings. This energy corresponds to the chi that EFT aims to harmonize.

Energy Meridians. The presence of the energy meridians is confirmed through the recently discovered Bonghan channels, which are physical channels of blood and lymph arranged in a pattern that corresponds to the meridians' layout.

The Influence of Mind on Matter. Recent studies prove that thought can change the physical components of the brain, the nervous system, the body organs, and even the genes within the cells. This means a lot to EFT because it affirms the power of thought to change what people feel and become. Quantum physics discoveries also strengthen the claim that people's thoughts change the reality they experience, which is an important idea in EFT.

What Skeptics Say

Some are quick to dismiss EFT as pseudoscience and quackery since it doesn't conform to what has already been studied by physics, biology, biochemistry, and other established sciences. These skeptics assume that EFT only works because of the mind's suggestibility and not because EFT is inherently effective. This may or may not be the case; it's hard to tell because EFT is still in its early stages and it deals with a lot of things that are currently beyond scientific measurements. However, the body of evidence proving that EFT works is constantly growing despite the criticisms against it. It may only be a matter of time when the processes behind EFT can be fully analyzed and be finally accepted as a legitimate and science-backed therapy.

Chapter 3: The Body's Energy System and the Tapping Points

EFT Tapping is a therapy that integrates knowledge from various fields of knowledge such as energy manipulation, psychology, hypnosis, and more. The main principle behind EFT is that energy affects people profoundly. By influencing how it runs through the body, people also modify the quality of their experiences.

Simply put, EFT tapping clears out the energy channels of the body, which the Chinese call as meridians. These are similar to blood vessels because they nourish every part of the individual, but unlike physical arteries and veins, meridians also affect the health of his emotions, mind, and soul.

A Brief Look at the Meridians

Meridians course throughout the body and serve as tunnels of subtle energy. There are two main energy types: yang and yin. They are polar opposites and complement each other – yang represents strength, forcefulness, and heat while yin symbolizes suppleness, fluidity, and coolness. EFT deals with these forces as well as other distinct energies. Each meridian is associated to a major organ but they affect the entire individual energetically.

Yin Meridians in the Arms

Lung meridian (LU). L1 to L11 travels from shoulder to the thumb. It influences the lungs, the throat and stomach.

Heart Meridian (H, HT or HE). H1 to H9 travels from the underarm to the hands' little fingers, but the meridian also includes points in the heart and the gut.

Pericardium meridian (PC or P). The pericardium meridian's 9 points traverse the center of the arm and ends within the chest.

Yang Meridians in the Arms

Large intestine meridian (LI or CO). This meridian has 20 points from the index finger and rises up through the arm, traverses the shoulders and curves up to the face below the nose.

Small intestine Meridian (SI). The small intestine meridian (S1-S19) travels up the pinky fingers up to the arm and the sides of the face. The small intestines are also connected to this meridian even though it's not physically linked to the rest of the points.

Triple burner meridian (a.ka. triple burner, triple warmer or San Jiao - TB, TW, or SJ). It is mostly found behind the body, specifically at the back of the neck, shoulders and arms, but a portion extends to the sides of the face near the ears. 23 points cover this meridian.

Yin Meridians in the Legs

Spleen meridian (SP). The spleen meridian winds up from the toe and reaches up to the stomach and spleen. It ends at SP 21 located near the armpit.

Kidney meridian (KI or K). The kidney meridian commences at the sole of the foot and rises up the center of the body. It ends at point 27 near the chest.

Liver Meridian (LV or LR). This has 14 points in all, with LV 1 starting on the side of the foot's big toe and ends up within the liver.

Yang Meridians in the Legs

Stomach Meridian. The stomach meridian (ST)'s starting point is found under the eye then diverges upward to the side of the head and downward through the stomach, the legs and ending at the toes. It contains 45 points.

Bladder Meridian (BL or UB). The bladder meridian is located mostly within the back. It starts at the corners of the eyes, climbs up to the crown of the head, and falls along the midline of the body to end at the feet. This makes up 67 points in all.

Gallbladder Merdian. The Gallblader meridian (GB) has 44 points that begin from the side of the head, wind down the body's sides, and ends at the toes.

Governing Vessel/Du (GV). The governing vessel meridian is the main passage of yang energy spanning 28 points in all. It starts from the perineum, goes up through the person's back, loops along the head, and ends within the upper part of a person's mouth.

Conception Vessel/Ren (CV). The conception vessel meridian harbors yin energy and is said to nourish the genitals and blood. It also begins from the perineum then rises to CV 24 beneath the chin.

√ EFT Points

These points are said to be the crucial locations where tapping can produce effects that reverberate throughout the body's meridians. Percussive movements on these locations shake off congestions formed by stress, unstable emotions, and other kinds of destructive energy. The following list details the different tapping points in the body (See EFT points diagram below):

1. **Eyebrow point**, which is located closest to the inside end of your left eyebrow, located on either side of the nose. Do make sure though, that you do not go down to your nose's bridge.

   EB – (UB 2) Found near the beginning of the urinary bladder meridian and the stomach meridian.

2. **Side-of-the-eye point**, which is located closest to the outside end of your right eye. This is the bone on the outside corner of your eye. Make sure that you do not poke your eyeball. If you suddenly notice that your vision started to become blurred or you see a flash of light or darkness, it means that the incorrect spot is being tapped.

   SE - Side of Eye (GB 1) The beginning of the gall bladder meridian, located near the end of the triple burner meridian and the small intestine meridian.

3. **Under-the-eye point**, which is located on your left cheekbone just under your pupil. If you have sinusitis, you can choose to tap very lightly.

UE - Under the Eye (St 1). The starting point of the stomach meridian.

4. **Under-the-nose point**, which is located exactly between your nose and your upper lip.

   UN - Under the Nose (GV 26). This is where the large intestine meridian ends and meets the governing meridian

5. **Under-the-mouth point**, which is located on the dip that connects your chin and lower lip.

   CH - Chin (CV 24). The end of the conception vessel and links to the start of the stomach meridian under the eyes.

6. **Collarbone point**, which is located exactly where your collarbone and your sternum meet.

   CB - Collar Bone (Ki 27). The end point of the kidney meridian.

7. **Under-the-arm point**, which is located on the side of your body that is nearer the back side than the front – around four inches down your armpit. If you poke your fingers in the area, you will find it as the tenderest part. To be that you are tapping on the right spot, use all your four fingers when you tap on the under-the-arm point.

   UA - UnderArm (Sp 21). Where the spleen meridian ends.

8. **Top-of-the-head point**, which is the peak or highest point on the top of your head.

EFT makes use of tapping techniques and other psychological methods to deal with energetic imbalances. These activities achieve specific beneficial results that vary from curing phobias to promoting a healthy lifestyle.

√ EFT Points Diagram

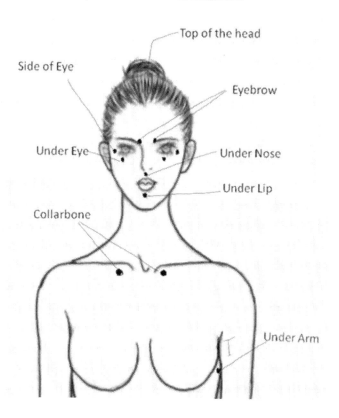

Chapter 4: The Four Steps of Basic EFT Application

One of the attractions of EFT is that it is very easy to perform and yet its effects are very significant. EFT skills can both be easily learned and be easily done by anybody, anywhere. As we have mentioned earlier, there are several ways you could use EFT and there are distinct details for each specific application. In relation to the many ways that it could be used, EFT can be compared to a knife – a simple tool that anybody can use anywhere. However, how the knife is actually used greatly depends on the particular person who uses it.

An ordinary person can use a knife to cut vegetables and meat while cooking. An artist can use it to create beautiful woodworks. The same knife used by different people creates different things. It doesn't mean that the knife is more useful to the ordinary person. It also doesn't mean that the artist is the only one who could use the knife properly. In other words, both the ordinary person and the artist could become better when it comes to using a knife. Both could take further studies or undergo additional training to become more skilled.

EFT acts in the same way. It is a very simple and flexible tool and its results will vary depending on who is actually employing it. Like any other ability, it is ideal that you become highly skilled in the basics first prior to attempting more complex tasks. If you attempt and choose to do complicated steps right away, you may just end up frustrated and you may decide to completely forget about using EFT. Continuing with our analogy of the knife, you should first study the mechanical uses of the knife (such as cutting) because you can use it in creating works of art.

I hope that you are not discouraged by this, because the basic "recipe" of EFT that you will learn here is incredibly valuable. Even if you do not progress to more advanced skills, the basic technique could already help you achieve astonishing results. Just always remember that you need to learn how to walk before you could learn how to run.

Like all endeavors, it will take some time before you could finally master EFT. You just need to remember that the more you practice the emotional freedom technique and the more information you learn about effective EFT practice, the higher your chances of succeeding. People who have gained quite a mastery of the emotional freedom technique still continue to set aside enough time for them to further sharpen their skills and to gain more information. If you notice that EFT is not working for you, take it as an opportunity to go a little further and a chance to become better at applying the emotional freedom technique.

√ The basic EFT "recipe"

The basic EFT "recipe" consists of the following four steps, which will be discussed in detail in the next chapters:

Step 0 - **Drink water**

Step 1 - **Tune in and rate**

Step 2 – **Clearing of psychological reversal**

Step 3 – **Tap**

Step 4 – **Tune in and re-rate**

27

√ The basic EFT Script

A **tapping script** is a simple phrase that is said repeatedly while tapping a particular point in the body. This is a way to let your system know what issue you are addressing. In creating the phrase, two goals must be met. The first line should acknowledge the issue that you want to address and the second line should be about self-acceptance in spite of the problem mentioned in the first line.

The following statement is a typical formula:

"In spite of (state your problem), I accept myself completely."

Take note that the problem statement must be **specific**. It must focus on **your very own** issue and not on someone else's issue. EFT aims at our personal involvement in the matter not anyone else's. Consider the following sample statements:

Being overweight:
"In spite of being overweight, I accept myself completely."

It is important to note that a negative language must be used to highlight the problem. This negativity is the cause of the energy disruptions that EFT aims to clear. Positive thinking does little in the overall effectiveness of tapping.

Having a script reprograms your mind to accept yourself just the way you are. This is a powerful way to restore your self-confidence and detach yourself from any negative misconceptions.

The Preparatory Steps

√ Step Zero

Humans are basically made up of 60 to 80 percent water (although the specific percentage depends on a person's age). The water within our bodies is actually what binds our whole body as one. When our body is without water, we could easily perish.

Another important feature of water is that it is an amazing conductor of energy. It is actually the structure of water that holds the body's many different parts together. Those structures are also the trails wherein the energy information of the communication system of the human body passes through. If our bodies lack water, the healing information will have no trail to pass through. In the book "Energy Medicine in Therapeutics and Human Performance", James Oschman wrote that a five-percent increase in water consumption could boost our bodies' ability to pass along those healing information by roughly five million times.

Generally, constant hydration is one of the secrets to a healthy overall wellbeing. Moreover, this is the reason why drinking water is a critical step in EFT. If your body is suffering from dehydration, you can almost expect that EFT will not really work. Therefore, if you didn't drink water in the past two hours, you should not start your tapping exercise. Simply put, you should drink water before following any of the other steps discussed in this book.

√ __Step One__ – Tune In and Rate

For Physical Illnesses

It is ideal to always have a pen and paper every time you perform EFT. Now that you are ready to begin the first step, it is important for you to know what "tuning in" means when working with EFT. When it comes to physical illnesses, it means that you will need to pay close attention to the source of the pain you are experiencing to make the pain be fully encompassed by your energy system. As we have discussed earlier, pain, illnesses, or a failure to heal are all caused by a disruption in the energy system of your body. In order for you to work in eliminating that disruption, you need to focus your energy.

Imagine when you want to clean all the dirty dishes in your home. You will only be able to do the actual cleaning after you have gathered all the dirty dishes found in different places in the house and put them in the sink. This is the same concept when working with EFT. You need to put everything you want to work on in your "sink" by focusing on the issue or concern that bothers you. The rationale behind focusing or tuning is that we often do not pay enough attention to the signals that our body gives us.

For instance, you could actually have sore feet, but you do not really feel the pain radiating from your feet until you go home at night and take off your shoes. Throughout the day, you are so used to tuning out such pains because you are more focused on your tasks. However, as soon as you get home, you feel all the pain because they get your undivided attention.

When you want to use EFT to heal any physical illness, you need to channel your focus on the particular area that you want to heal – that basically comprises the process of tuning in. Unlike the pain in your feet that you involuntarily felt when you got home, the first step in the EFT process will require you to intentionally focus on your aches and pains. You can do this by closing your eyes and taking a deep breath as you inspect your whole body for any tightness or physical pain. Choose any of the pains that you feel as your primary focus.

Since you are just beginning to practice EFT, it is ideal that you select a persistent pain that you have been feeling for several months or even years. As we have discussed earlier, you will more likely to succeed if you choose a simpler task to accomplish during your first try.

After you have selected one pain or tension, begin to ask yourself questions such as:

- Where is the exact location of my pain? (your answer should be something specific, like this – right shin starting from just below the knee, down until just above the feet).

- How immense is the pain that I feel? (again be specific, say something descriptive like – around 12 inches long that is as thin as a pencil).

- If I can picture the pain, what color will it be? Just try your instincts. Don't think too hard on this.

- What type of pain am I feeling – sharp, blunt, pulsing?

- What emotion best describes that pain that I'm feeling?

- On a scale of zero to ten (zero being "no pain" and ten being "worst pain"), how will I rate my pain? The answer to this question will be the rating that you will use as a baseline.

Jot down your answers on the paper that you prepared. If you cannot think of any an answer to any question, just skip it. However, do not skip a question just because you think it is weird. Always keep in mind that the more detail you have about your pain, the higher your chances of making EFT work for you.

How to be specific for your EFT Tapping Therapy?

Specific statement has a much greater chance of being accomplished than a general one.

To set a specific Tapping EFT script you can answer these questions:

1. Who is involved?

2. What do I want to accomplish?

3. Where: Identify a location.

4. When: establish a time frame.

5. What are the specific reasons of the problem?

6. What are the specific reasons of my problem?

7. What is the specific emotion?

8. How will I know when it is accomplished?

9. Can your goals be measurable?

10. What exactly are you thinking or telling yourself?
For Emotional Problems

Tuning in to your emotional problems is more complicated than tuning in to a physical pain because it is sometimes harder to be specific enough. So, let us just use Gary Craig's analogy of a table in identifying an emotional "pain" to tune in to. Think of your emotional problem (fear, helplessness, desperation, or fury) as a tabletop. A tabletop requires at least three legs to stand upright as a table. Your emotional problem is the same. You have bad memories that act as the legs of your emotional problem. For instance, if you are afraid of speaking in public, the following memories may have become the legs of your fear:

- You spoke in front of adults as a little child and you were vehemently reprimanded because of it.

- You presented a project in school and heard your classmates snickering.

- You gave a speech and forgot your lines, and so everyone laughed.

EFT is not that effective in destroying your "tabletop", but it can definitely help you in destroying each of the legs one at a time. If we look at the above examples, you could choose to work on your problem with being laughed at. The specific pain that you would focus on (which you will use in the next steps) can be stated as "feeling defensive and self-conscious when I hear other people laughing at me". After you have tuned it, you could use the same scale we used with physical illnesses.

Still, remember to rate yourself based on the emotions you feel when you recall the memory now and not when the event actually happened. Write your emotional pain and its corresponding rating on your paper or notebook.

√ <u>**Step Two**</u> – **Clearing of Psychological Reversal**

It was Roger Callahan M.D who invented the phrase "Psychological Reversal" while he was building Thought Field Therapy (or TFT), which was a predecessor of EFT. Dr. Roger Callahan noted that no matter how much tapping a certain person does following the standard procedures of TFT, no healing was achieved. Aside from that, whatever physical illness or emotional problem the person was experiencing persisted. He then was able to come to the conclusion that TFT was not effective in certain people because their bodies are "psychologically reversed".

This is a condition wherein the energetic field that surrounds the specific area where the issue occurs is reversed. For you to better understand this concept, imagine that our bodies consist of energetic fields that act like magnets. When our bodies are in their normal or healthy status, it means that energy flowing inside our bodies go from the top of our heads down to the bottom of our feet (north to south).

When a person becomes psychologically reversed, it means that the energy flowing inside his or her body goes from the bottom of the feet up to the top of the head. When this occurs, it is virtually impossible to heal the mind and body of any illness. This is the reason why step two is very critical. Do not worry though, because clearing your psychological reversal is quite simple to accomplish – and it doesn't come with any negative effect.

√ To perform step two, tap the area "karate chop" (See karate chop point diagram below).

You may choose the hand, which feels more comfortable for you. Use the four fingers of your dominant hand to tap on the dotted area of the other hand. Continue tapping until you have finished saying all the following statements:

- **Although I have this pain on {insert your own pain}, I still love and fully accept myself.**

- **Although I have this pain on {insert your own pain}, I forgive myself for whatever I have done to contribute to the pain.**

- **Although I have this pain on {insert your own pain}, I forgive the other people who have added to my pain**

- **Although I have this pain on {insert your own pain}, I will forever love and fully accept myself.**

Make sure that you say the statements aloud and energetically, as if what the statements mean are actually true even though you do not fully believe them. I know it may sometimes be difficult to say something that you do not truly believe in. However, just trust in the process and you will eventually feel in your heart that you are starting to believe those statements.

√ Karate Chop Point Diagram

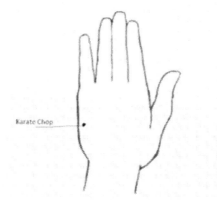

Karate Chop

The Final Critical Steps

√ <u>Step 3</u>: Start Tapping (Tap)

After you have cleared your psychological reversal, you are now ready to start tapping your index and middle fingers on the following points of your body:

Here are **the steps in tapping** which will make use of the same four statements from the previous step:

1. Tap on the first point while saying the four statements. Continue tapping until you have said all statements.

2. Go to and tap the second point while saying the four statements.

3. Repeat the tapping and the statements until you have completed all eight points.

4. After you have finished, inhale and exhale deeply.

Drink just enough water.

√ <u>Step 4</u> – Tune in and Re-rate

This step is the simplest of all. Before you start, inhale and exhale deeply. Also, take another sip of water. When you are ready, tune in to the point of pain again and ask the following questions:

- Did the intensity of the pain decrease, increase, or stay the same?

- Did the pain move to another location, or did it spread to several spots?

- Was the "texture" or the kind of pain altered? (for example, it was previously a sharp pain, which now has become just a dull pain).

- Did any image, vision, or thought entered your mind while you were tapping the different body points? Were there any memory or person you remembered? If you answered "yes" to any of these questions, whatever entered your mind might be connected to the pain that you are currently working on.

- Rate how your pain feels now using the same scale of zero to ten.

Part 2
Get Your Food Control Back

Tapping for Weight Loss

Chapter 5: Weight Loss and the Reality of Emotions

Eating Your Heart Out?

Who doesn't have a love affair with food? The human brain is wired to derive great pleasure from eating. It fills us up and fuels our bodies so we can adequately complete the tasks of the day. A hearty stew silences a growling stomach and a velvety chocolate bar melts in our mouth along with our worries. More than providing nourishment, food has also become a source of comfort especially when dealing with stress.

Emotional eating or stress eating is a coping mechanism that refers to the tendency of people to eat as a way of dealing with tough situations. The sugary taste of chocolate chip cookies or the texture of a well-cooked steak provides that much needed momentary escape from a draining situation.

A lot of factors come into play when dealing with weight gain and obesity; and often times the main problem runs deeper than the skin's surface. Negative emotions such as anxiety, anger and loneliness also trigger excessive eating habits. People who fail to deal with the root cause of these emotions often find themselves in an endless battle with weight gain even after months of dieting.

An effective weight loss plan begins with identifying the root cause of your negative emotions. It helps you focus on the real problem and how you actually deal with them. A simple way of doing this is to document your emotions.

In the next few days, take a moment to write down what you think and feel before you eat. The key here is to be honest and write as much detail as possible. This exercise will help you become more aware of your eating habits; enabling you to recognize the times when you are most likely to eat due to your emotions.

The effectiveness of this method has been proven in a 2008 study conducted by the University of Kentucky. The results revealed that most people are more likely to choose low-calorie foods when they are mindful of their feelings.

The Role of EFT in Effective Weight Loss

The subconscious mind is the only thing that comes between you and your ideal body. It sounds quite surreal but it's true. All of us are born with a clean slate and as we grow old, a lot of factors and external events mold our concept of self. For most people with weight problems a lot of their emotional issues pile up and are left unresolved either consciously or unconsciously, leading them to their struggle. The only way to get out of the endless cycle of depression, self-loathing, and food addiction is to acknowledge these feelings and address them properly. This is where EFT comes into the picture.

As discussed in the first chapter, EFT is a two-step process that begins with identifying an emotional issue that makes a person overeats. In some cases, a person can easily identify the root cause of their struggle.

However, there are people, battling with weight issues for a long time, who may find it difficult to pinpoint the cause due to the accumulation of hurts in past experiences.

In any case, any unresolved issue can be resurfaced by asking yourself the following questions and answering them as honestly as you can:

**What do you think is the major
cause of stress in your life at this point?**
(Is it finances, relationships, career, etc.?)

**What are you going through when the
issue started?**
(Bankruptcy, career shift, misfortune, etc)

**What is the one complaint that you
always rant about?**
(People are mean to me, I never get what
I deserve, I don't feel welcome, etc)

Your answers to these questions should reveal an obvious point that you have to deal with.

But if a lot of issues resurface, the best thing to do is to choose **one** just to get started. Emotional issues are often interrelated. Addressing one problem can potentially lead to finding ways to address the other issues.

As an emotional issue is made known, tapping on it should make you feel relieved from any physical discomfort.

Take note that in most cases, 'the one' issue is not easily identified. Expect to address more than one issue before completely resolving your weight problem.

Mirror, Mirror, on the Wall,
Who's the Slimmest of them All?

The Mirror Exercise is one of the most effective ways to eliminate negative emotions and beliefs about your self-image. It typically takes 10 to 15 minutes of quiet time, repeated twice a day. The recommended times are during sunrise and sunset. In case these times are inconvenient for you, you can find two other times when you can be alone.

The following steps describe the whole process of this popular self-acceptance and healing method:

1. In a room that is not too hot or too cold, stand in front of a full length mirror, completely naked. This is your opportunity to see your whole self. Place your feet, shoulder-width apart such that if a straight line is drawn from the outer edge of your shoulder downwards, it should touch the edge of your foot. Divide your weight evenly on each foot.

2. Spend a few minutes taking in your whole reflection then turn your attention to your forehead, focus your sight at the point that is exactly between your reflection's eyes.

3. For the duration of the exercise, say the following words repeatedly to yourself: "Even if I have a problem with (insert emotional issue), I accept myself completely. I love myself, just the way I am." For greater benefit, translate this statement into your own language.

4. Put your hands together, palms pushed against each other in front of you. As you do this, be aware of the pressure in your palms and in your upper body.

5. Close your eyes. Inhale. Imagine your breath coming in through the top of your head, filling your center, and then leaving from the soles of your feet. Exhale. This is one breath cycle. In the next cycle imagine the reverse; your breath comes into the soles of your feet, filling your center, and then leaving from the top of your head. Focus on the sound of your breath as it goes through your body.

6. As you exhale, release any negative thought, impression or feeling that comes to mind and use the inhaled air to fill the emptied space created upon the release of a thought.

Initially, you may find it difficult to focus on your breath due to the tons of things that flood your mind. Don't worry. With constant practice and a conscious effort to calm the mind, you will be able to master this technique over time.

The main benefit of this exercise is self-acceptance. Seeing your whole body in the mirror makes you aware of your imperfections and positive qualities. Listening to your breathing helps you attune yourself with your innermost thoughts.

This process enables you to identify your thinking pattern.

By releasing any negative thoughts or misconceptions about yourself, you are able to clear your mind of worries and anxieties. Self-awareness increases as you constantly practice this exercise.

Being mindful of your thoughts helps you direct your actions towards better habits.

By agreeing to do this activity, you are taking courage to see yourself as you are. Keeping an open mind is important as it will help you release any inhibitions that may impede your healing.

Chapter 6: The Basic Recipe for Weight Loss

√ The Basic Recipe for Weight Loss

The basic EFT "recipe" consists of the following four steps, which will be discussed in detail in the next chapters:

Step 0 - Drink water

Step 1 - Tune in and rate

Close your eyes. Take a deep breath as you inspect your whole body for any tightness or physical pain. On a scale of zero to ten (zero being "no pain" and ten being "worst pain"), how will I rate my emotional pain?

The answer to this question will be the rating that you will use as a baseline. Keep in mind that the more detail you have about your pain, the higher your chances of making EFT work for you.

Step 2 – Clearing of psychological reversal

Psychologically reversed is a condition wherein the energetic field that surrounds the specific area where the issue occurs is reversed.

To perform psychological reversal for weight loss issues, tap the area with red dots in the picture below ("karate point"). You may choose the hand, which feels more comfortable for you. Use the four fingers of your dominant hand to tap on the dotted area of the other hand. Tap about 7 seconds for each statement.

Continue tapping until you have finished saying all the following statements:

- **In spite of being overweight, I accept myself completely, I still love and fully accept myself.**

- **In spite of being overweight, I forgive myself for whatever I have done to contribute to the pain.**

- **In spite of being overweight, I forgive the other people who have added to my pain**

- **In spite of being overweight, I will forever love and fully accept myself.**

Repeat psychological reversal three times. Make sure that you say the statements aloud and energetically, as if what the statements mean are actually true even though you do not fully believe them.

I know it may sometimes be difficult to say something that you do not truly believe in. However, just **trust in the process** and you will eventually feel in your heart that you are starting to believe those statements. However, you can say the statements **silently** or by heart as you breathe.

Step 3 – Tap

Here are the steps in tapping. Tap about 7 seconds on each of the points.

1. Tap on the first point while saying the four statements. Continue tapping until you have said all statements.

2. Go to and tap the second point while saying the four statements.

3. Repeat the tapping and the statements until you have completed all eight points.

4. After you have finished, inhale and exhale deeply.

5. Drink just enough water.

Start tapping your index and middle fingers on the tapping points of your body:

Eyebrow point, which is located closest to the inside end of your left eyebrow. Do make sure though, that you do not go down to your nose's bridge.

"In spite of being overweight, I still love
and fully accept myself."

"In spite of being overweight, I forgive myself
for whatever I have done to contribute to the pain."

"In spite of being overweight, I forgive the other
people who have added to my pain."

"In spite of being overweight, I will forever love
and fully accept myself."

Side-of-the-eye point, which is located closest to the outside end of your right eye. Make sure that you do not poke your eyeball. If you suddenly notice that your vision started to become blurred or you see a flash of light or darkness, it means that the incorrect spot is being tapped.

"In spite of being overweight, I still love
and fully accept myself."

"In spite of being overweight, I forgive myself
for whatever I have done to contribute to the pain."

"In spite of being overweight, I forgive
the other people who have added to my pain."

"In spite of being overweight, I will forever love
and fully accept myself."

<u>Under-the-eye point</u>, which is located on your left cheekbone just under your pupil. If you have sinusitis, you can choose to tap very lightly.

"In spite of being overweight, I still love
and fully accept myself."

"In spite of being overweight, I forgive myself
for whatever I have done to contribute to the pain."

"In spite of being overweight, I forgive the other
people who have added to my pain."

"In spite of being overweight, I will forever love
and fully accept myself."

<u>Under-the-nose point</u>, which is located exactly between your nose and your upper lip.

"In spite of being overweight, I still love
and fully accept myself."

"In spite of being overweight, I forgive myself
for whatever I have done to contribute to the pain."

"In spite of being overweight, I forgive the other
people who have added to my pain."

"In spite of being overweight, I will forever love
and fully accept myself."

Under-the-mouth point, which is located on the dip that
connects your chin and lower lip.

"In spite of being overweight, I still love
and fully accept myself."

"In spite of being overweight, I forgive myself
for whatever I have done to contribute to the pain."

"In spite of being overweight, I forgive the other
people who have added to my pain."

"In spite of being overweight, I will forever love
and fully accept myself."

Collarbone point, which is located exactly where your
collarbone and your sternum meet.

"In spite of being overweight, I still love
and fully accept myself."

"In spite of being overweight, I forgive myself
for whatever I have done to contribute to the pain."

"In spite of being overweight, I forgive the other
people who have added to my pain."

"In spite of being overweight, I will forever
love and fully accept myself."

Under-the-arm point, which is located on the side of your
body that is nearer the back side than the front – around four
inches down your armpit. If you poke your fingers in the area,
you will find it as the most tender part. To be that you are
tapping on the right spot, use all your four fingers when you tap
on the under-the-arm point.

"In spite of being overweight, I still love
and fully accept myself."

"In spite of being overweight, I forgive myself
for whatever I have done to contribute to the pain."

"In spite of being overweight, I forgive the other
people who have added to my pain."

"In spite of being overweight, I will forever love
and fully accept myself."

Top-of-the-head point, which is the peak or highest point on
the top of your head.

"In spite of being overweight, I still love
and fully accept myself."

"In spite of being overweight, I forgive myself
for whatever I have done to contribute to the pain."

"In spite of being overweight, I forgive the other people who have added to my pain."

"In spite of being overweight, I will forever love and fully accept myself."

Step 4 – Tune in and re-rate

Inhale and exhale deeply. Also, take another sip of water. When you are ready, tune in to the point of emotional pain again and ask the following questions:

- Did the intensity of the pain decrease, increase, or stay the same?

- Did any image, vision, or thought entered your mind while you were tapping the different body points?

- Were there any memory or person you remembered?

If you answered "yes" to any of these questions, whatever entered your mind might be connected to the pain that you are currently working on.

Rate how you feel now using the same scale of zero to ten.

Chapter 7: Taming Hunger Pangs

Food and Emotions

A lot of us live by the belief that: we live to eat. People eat to socialize, to get rid of boredom, and even bond with long lost loved ones. Eating is also a way of responding to emotions such as anxiety.

There is a reason why comfort food is even considered a food category and that emotional eating is a type of appetite. The pleasure derived from eating provides a temporary relief from challenging and stressful experiences we encounter each day.

There's nothing wrong with giving in to our cravings from time to time. Yet, there is much sense in the old saying that too much of something is bad. Emotional eating is a habit that can lead to a variety of health problems.

Imagine what happens every time you feel bummed out, and treat yourself to a big bar of sweet, enticing chocolate. What do you get in return?

A fleeting moment of happiness, coupled with a raging blood sugar and a ton of health problems in the long run. Problems are always a part of life. And the best way to deal with it is to face it head on.

We Why Crave

Associate professor Heather Hausenblas, Ph. D., from the University of Florida says that foods that are starchy, sugary or fatty taste delicious and the body recognizes that. As you chew a soft, warm, fudge brownie, a series of chemical reactions occur in the body that ultimately boosts the serotonin levels. Higher serotonin levels in the body makes a person feel more content albeit temporarily.

Vulnerability to cravings often occurs during stressful situations. Chronic stress elevates cortisol levels in the body. As a result, the body feels that it is going through a famine and in effect the cravings intensify. Suffering makes people feel deprived of a lot of things. Although a person's perspective on suffering significantly affects the way it is dealt with, most of us feel we deserve a break from all the negativity that a crisis or challenge brings.

This feeling pushes us to find ways to channel this negativity and for some, food is the best outlet. Because comfort food are often considered treats, a lot of us think that the more difficult a challenge is, the more we deserve to eat larger quantities of our favorite food.

The irony of it all is after consuming the food some people feel resentment towards the act.

Finding the root cause of your cravings can be done by being more mindful of your habits. Sometimes a simple habit such as skipping breakfast could lead to having food cravings. Ask yourself some of these questions to determine what may be the real cause of your cravings:

- Do you often skip meals, particularly breakfast?

- Do you find yourself eating lightly during breakfast?

- Do you often eat cereals, French toast or quick cooking oats for breakfast?

- Are you the type of person who drink lots of coffee with sugar each morning and then skip the actual meal, then compensate the hunger later with a pastry?

- Are you going through a rough patch in your life at this point?

- Do often feel stressed?

- Are you often deprived of sleep?

If you found yourself answering yes to most of these questions then chances are, you've set yourself up to have cravings each day.

Curbing Your Cravings with EFT

EFT is a powerful way to curb **binge eating**. However, if you've been tapping down your cravings and have not achieved the desired results, chances are, you've not dealt with the deeper problem.

Bingeing can also be a symptom of another issue you might not be aware of. Before grabbing a snack in between meals, take time to reflect on your feelings at the moment. Do you feel lonely, fearful or anxious? By doing this simple exercise, you will be able to identify what emotions trigger your hunger. Only then will you be able to make a concrete action about it.

The next time you find yourself just about to binge, do these simple tapping exercises:

√ Tapping before snacking

1. At the moment exactly before eating, say the following:

    **"I will eat this _____ (pizza, brownie, chip, etc)
    and nothing or no one will stop me. I accept the feelings
    that I have in me, right now at this moment."**

2.   Pause for a while, gently close your eyes and gradually tune into your body. Observe any sensation going through your body, its intensity and what kinds of emotion come up (regret, helplessness, boredom, etc)

3. Begin tapping on the stressful emotion (regret, helplessness, boredom, etc) by reciting the script:

**"In spite of (the stressful emotion you're experiencing),
I accept myself completely."**

Then proceed with the tapping sequence.
If you find that the emotion does not change in intensity, think of what the emotion reminds you of. You can then tap on that event.

Do this until you are able to pinpoint the root cause of your bingeing. (see **The Complete EFT Recipe for Binge Eating** at the end of this chapter)

Searching for Clues Using Your Imagination

When you experience craving, take a deep breath, shut your eyes and focus on the food that you're currently craving for. Picture how it looks. Relive its color, aroma. Feel its texture as you hold it and place it into your mouth. Savor its flavor. Take all the time you need. No rush. Recall your experience when eating this particular food.

As your imagination works to relive the experience you had when eating this food, identify the point in your body where you strongly feel the craving. Focus on this spot. Feel your heart and place your hand on it. Ask yourself honestly, the following questions:

Is there something that needs to be healed,
cleared or accepted? Is there a gap that remains
to be filled?

Be mindful of any insight that may come up. Each person treats food differently in response to the unique issues that have resulted from their own experiences. People who have a problem accepting themselves find comfort in snacking and see it as a way to validate their existence. Others who were abused in their younger years find overeating as a way to get bigger so that they could protect themselves from harm.

EFT is great way to curb any craving because it gives you the opportunity to get in touch with your inner self and identify your real snacking triggers. Be more open with yourself as you practice these methods.

√ The Complete EFT Recipe for Binge Eating

Step 0 - Drink water

Step 1 - Tune in and rate

Step 2 – Clearing of psychological reversal

Tap about 7 seconds for each statement on your karate point. Continue tapping until you have finished saying all the following statements:

- **In spite of my helplessness / boredom, etc, I still love and fully accept myself.**

- **In spite of my helplessness / boredom, etc, I forgive myself for whatever I have done to contribute to the pain.**

- **In spite of my helplessness / boredom, etc, I forgive the other people who have added to my pain**

- **In spite of my helplessness / boredom, etc, I will forever love and fully accept myself.**

Repeat psychological reversal three times.

Step 3 – Tap

Here are the steps in tapping. Repeat tapping about 7 seconds on each of the points.

Start tapping your index and middle fingers on the tapping points of your body:

<u>Eyebrow point</u>
"I accept my helplessness / boredom, etc"

<u>Side-of-the-eye point</u>
"I accept my helplessness / boredom, etc"

<u>Under-the-eye point</u>
"I accept my helplessness / boredom, etc"

<u>Under-the-nose point</u>
"I accept my helplessness / boredom, etc"

<u>Under-the-mouth point</u>
"I accept my helplessness / boredom, etc"

<u>Collarbone point</u>
"I accept my helplessness / boredom, etc"

<u>Under-the-arm point</u>
"I accept my helplessness / boredom, etc"

<u>Top-of-the-head point</u>
"I accept my helplessness / boredom, etc"

Step 4 – Tune in and re-rate

Chapter 8: Optimizing your Metabolism with EFT

√ Optimizing your Metabolism with EFT

Understanding how the body uses the food you eat is important especially when you want to shed some pounds. Metabolism is a natural process by which the body converts all that you eat into energy. It is a non-stop cycle that occurs in two steps. The first step, anabolism, involves the creation and storage of energy while the second step, catabolism, refers to the release of this energy. The endocrine system is responsible for keeping metabolism in control just like it does with cell growth and mood regulation.

While you can't command your metabolism to change at will, you can definitely influence it. You can decide what kinds of food you'll eat as well as its quantity. Your activity level also influences your metabolism. Ultimately, everything boils down to proper diet and regular exercise. Jillian Michaels, the Biggest Loser strength coach and author of the New York Times bestseller, Making the Cut, proposes three ways to boost metabolism:

- Remove anti-nutrients in your diet that activate your fat storing hormone.

- Restore foods that activate your fat loss hormones.

- Rebalance your food intake and energy levels to optimize your metabolism.

Removing Anti-nutrients from Your Diet

Processed foods are heaven sent for people on the go. Yet the convenience that it brings comes at a hefty price: your health. Get rid of the following the following items in your diet:

Hydrogenated fat – used by processed food manufacturers to keep cookies, chips and crackers fresh for a longer time; frequent consumption of hydrogenated fat increases your bad cholesterol levels while decreasing your good cholesterol levels.

Refined grains – such as white pasta, white rice, white bread have been stripped of the fiber, minerals and vitamins due to the removal of the bran and germ of the grain used to manufacture these products; easier to digest causing the blood sugar and insulin to spike.

High fructose corn syrup (HFCS) – it is the cheapest sweetener around that does nothing but boost the body's fat storing hormone.

Artificial sweeteners – same effect as HFCS.

Artificial flavoring and color – can potentially damage the body's natural biochemistry and inhibit metabolism.

Glutamates – known as flavor enhancers; it is a form of excitotoxin whereby excessive amounts in the body lead to brain cell damage.

Restoring these Foods in Your Meals

Previously, we got rid of the toxic food items in your diet. At this point, incorporating these food groups can repair your metabolism and restore hormonal balance in your body.

<u>Legumes</u> – beans are considered to have abundant amounts of soluble fibre that is key in controlling blood sugar; high in zinc and B vitamins that boost testosterone levels.

<u>Alliums</u> – such as garlic, onions, leeks, chives, shallots and scallions; this food group are considered as body detoxers since they combat free radicals that are present in your system.

<u>Berries</u> – contain anthocyanins that prevent insulin spikes that can lead to diabetes.

<u>Meat and eggs</u> – food sources that are rich in amino acids; protein increases the metabolic rate since they are harder to break down; as a result you feel full longer.

<u>Cruciferous veggies</u> – such as broccoli contain cancer fighting properties; the byproduct of ingesting these veggies is isothionate, a compound that eliminates carcinogens present in your system.

<u>Nuts and Seeds</u> - great protein sources that also prevent heart disease, diabetes and organ inflammation.

<u>Organic Dairy</u> – great source of calcium; sufficient levels of calcium in the body prevents the development of metabolic syndromes.

<u>Whole grains</u> – rich in phytochemicals and antioxidants

Rebalancing Your Diet and Energy

Now that you know what foods to avoid or include in your diet, let's revisit the concept of balance. Rebalancing your diet can significantly affect your hormone and metabolism. By eating at regular times of the day, your body is able to follow its natural rhythm and regularly execute its calorie-burning tasks.

Breakfast is indeed the most important meal of the day. Eating the morning meal jumpstarts your metabolism and keeps you up and running for the rest of the day. A lot of studies show that skipping breakfast induces cravings which are why a high percentage of breakfast skippers are more prone to diabetes and obesity as they age. Eating until you're full but not stuffed also leads to an optimized metabolism and a healthy body.

Managing your stress and rebalancing your energy are also crucial in boosting your metabolism. Avoid overworking your brain and underworking your body. Sleeping for at least 7 hours each night is necessary for hormonal balance. This is your body's opportunity to recover and repair the tissues and muscles that have been strained during the day. Less sleep makes you feel tired. To regain your energy, you tend to give in to any craving you have at the moment. And as you might have guessed, it only disrupts the hormone balance that you're aiming to achieve.

Exercise dramatically affects your metabolic process. The benefits of physical activity are endless: the release of fat-burning growth hormone; reduction of cortisol; increased sensitivity of your cells to insulin. A healthy dose of endorphins also result from exercise. This stuff keeps your mood positive and improves your overall reaction to stress.

√ Optimizing Your Metabolism with EFT

Your emotional connection with food makes EFT a valid method not just to curb cravings but also to optimize metabolism. Follow this simple exercise in your free time:

1. Ask yourself what percent you think your metabolism is functioning at this stage in your life. Don't think of an answer; allow a number to come to mind.

2. Recite the following lines for the first set of tapping:

   **"Even if my metabolism is only ___ percent,
   I fully accept and love my body as it is."**

3. On the second set of tapping say:

   **"I am releasing everything that slows me down
   and I fully accept and love my body as it is."**

4. On your third round of tapping say:

   **"I will repair everything that slows me down.
   I fully accept and love my body as it is."**

After the session, ask yourself again the percentage at which you metabolism is functioning. See if there's any improvement. If not, you can always repeat the process until healing takes place.

√ The Complete EFT Recipe for Optimizing Your Metabolism

The first set: tapping to optimize your metabolism

Step 0 - Drink water

Step 1 - Tune in and rate

Step 2 – Clearing of psychological reversal

Tap about 7 seconds for each statement on your karate point. Continue tapping until you have finished saying all the following statements:

**"Even if my metabolism is only ___ percent,
I fully accept and love my body as it is."**

Repeat psychological reversal <u>three</u> times.

Step 3 – Tap

Here are the steps in tapping. Repeat tapping about 7 seconds on each of the points.

Start tapping your index and middle fingers on the tapping points of your body:

Eyebrow point
"Even if my metabolism is only ___ percent, I fully accept and love my body as it is"

Side-of-the-eye point
"Even if my metabolism is only ___ percent, I fully accept and love my body as it is"

Under-the-eye point
"Even if my metabolism is only ___ percent, I fully accept and love my body as it is"

Under-the-nose point
"Even if my metabolism is only ___ percent, I fully accept and love my body as it is"

Under-the-mouth point
"Even if my metabolism is only ___ percent, I fully accept and love my body as it is"

Collarbone point
"Even if my metabolism is only ___ percent, I fully accept and love my body as it is"

Under-the-arm point
"Even if my metabolism is only ___ percent, I fully accept and love my body as it is"

Top-of-the-head point
"Even if my metabolism is only ___ percent, I fully accept and love my body as it is"

Step 4 – Tune in and re-rate

The second set: tapping to optimize your metabolism

Step 0 - Drink water

Step 1 - Tune in and rate

Step 2 – Clearing of psychological reversal

Tap about 7 seconds for each statement on your karate point. Continue tapping until you have finished saying all the following statements:

"Even if I am not releasing everything that slows me down, I fully accept and love my body as it is."

Repeat psychological reversal <u>three</u> times.

Step 3 – Tap

Here are the steps in tapping. Repeat tapping about 7 seconds on each of the points.

Start tapping your index and middle fingers on the tapping points of your body:

<u>Eyebrow point</u>
"I am releasing everything that slows me down and I fully accept and love my body as it is."

Side-of-the-eye point

"I am releasing everything that slows me down and I fully accept and love my body as it is."

Under-the-eye point

"I am releasing everything that slows me down and I fully accept and love my body as it is."

Under-the-nose point

"I am releasing everything that slows me down and I fully accept and love my body as it is."

Under-the-mouth point

"I am releasing everything that slows me down and I fully accept and love my body as it is."

Collarbone point

"I am releasing everything that slows me down and I fully accept and love my body as it is."

Under-the-arm point

"I am releasing everything that slows me down and I fully accept and love my body as it is."

Top-of-the-head point

"I am releasing everything that slows me down and I fully accept and love my body as it is."

Step 4 – Tune in and re-rate

The third set: tapping to optimize your metabolism

Step 0 - Drink water

Step 1 - Tune in and rate

Step 2 – Clearing of psychological reversal

Tap about 7 seconds for each statement on your karate point. Continue tapping until you have finished saying all the following statements:

**"Even if everything slows me down,
I fully accept and love my body as it is."**

Repeat psychological reversal <u>three</u> times.

Step 3 – Tap

Here are the steps in tapping. Repeat tapping about 7 seconds on each of the points.

Start tapping your index and middle fingers on the tapping points of your body:

<u>Eyebrow point</u>
**"I will repair everything that slows me down.
I fully accept and love my body as it is."**

Side-of-the-eye point

"I will repair everything that slows me down.
I fully accept and love my body as it is."

Under-the-eye point

"I will repair everything that slows me down.
I fully accept and love my body as it is."

Under-the-nose point

"I will repair everything that slows me down.
I fully accept and love my body as it is."

Under-the-mouth point

"I will repair everything that slows me down.
I fully accept and love my body as it is."

Collarbone point

"I will repair everything that slows me down.
I fully accept and love my body as it is."

Under-the-arm point

"I will repair everything that slows me down.
I fully accept and love my body as it is."

Top-of-the-head point

"I will repair everything that slows me down.
I fully accept and love my body as it is."

Step 4 – Tune in and re-rate

Chapter 9: Addressing Self-Acceptance with EFT

The process of losing weight is not just a physical change. It also entails going through emotional and at times spiritual changes to achieve the overall well-being that you desire. That said, self-acceptance is a crucial characteristic that might solely predict the success of your weight loss plans. It is actually the first step in your journey to a better self.

Self-acceptance is a pervasive issue around the world. It often stems from our habit of noticing the good in people and ignoring our strengths. A lot factors cultivate this mentality among individuals. It could be a tough childhood, less supportive parents, living in a culture of low self-esteem.

While we cannot change our past experiences, the way we react to situations today can change our future. Yes, you hold the key to self-acceptance.

If you acknowledge yourself and accept you as you are, you will feel more empowered to do things. You will be able to focus on your strengths and use your skills to gain advantage in life.

A positive self-image encourages you to be your best all the time. A positive self-image encourages you to maintain a healthy lifestyle.

Addressing Self-Acceptance with EFT

The first step is to decide that you will be happy with yourself despite your frustrations and limitations. Happiness is a choice and having a positive mind at the start will jumpstart your motivation to improve. The next step is to create a list of the things that you don't accept about yourself and apply EFT to them. Proceed by creating set-up statements for each item.

For example:

Finishing a bag of chips in one sitting

**"Even if I have just finished a bag of chips in one sitting,
I fully and wholeheartedly accept myself."**

**"Even if I am munching on a bag of chips instead of doing work,
I fully and wholeheartedly accept myself."**

**"Even if I won't be going anywhere with my current attitude,
I fully and wholeheartedly accept myself.f"**

**"In spite of my fear of being laughed at,
I accept myself completely."**

Timid people who regularly apply EFT on these irrational thoughts have felt that they are more empowered to deal with their problems head on; you should experience this benefit too.

Learn to accept your weaknesses and be empowered to tackle your weight issues with confidence.

Part 3
Tapping for Wealth

Tapping for Financial Abundance

Chapter 10: Money and your Internal Beliefs about Wealth and Financial Abundance

Money is the root of all evil...trees don't grow money...there will always be a limit to how much you can earn in your lifetime...These are probably some of the words you uttered to yourself at some point in your life. These statements reflect your internal beliefs about wealth and financial abundance which means you were harboring limiting money beliefs in your subconscious and it usually happens when we are at a losing end.

Sigmund Freud once likened the conscious mind to the tip of an iceberg and the subconscious is the submerged bigger part of the iceberg which means that there are more things happening within the subconscious that cannot be explained by science compared to our conscious state. Such analogy reflects that there is a vast power hiding behind our beliefs and subconscious.

Our beliefs are not always based on facts and truth instead, they are often influenced by what we have been taught since our formative years, and based on what we have seen, heard and experienced in our life. The beliefs that we have right now towards money clearly dictate our state of well-being and financial health. The people around us and the environment we live in greatly affect our internal beliefs about financial abundance and wealth.

For example, a person who was raised in a poor environment where money is scarce and luxury is just dream sees money in a different light compared to someone who was raised in a well-to-do environment where everything is provided in an instant and money is plentiful. Similarly, if two persons both came from a poor background, their education and upbringing will affect their beliefs and attitude towards money. If the other person was taught that money can be earned and if he believes that he can be rich despite his poor background, that person clearly demonstrate a higher possibility of being successful in life compared to the other person who have already given up and resigned to the unfortunate life he's currently in.

It is natural for us to make limiting statements and have limiting beliefs which are often manifested in the decisions we make. These limiting beliefs however, should not define how you should live your life. If we remain in the dark, these limiting beliefs will be powerful enough to drag us down. The good news is we can reframe and change our internal beliefs about money to be able to attract wealth and financial abundance into our life.

First, we need to be aware about our limiting money beliefs. This is possible if we can go back in time and recall the times when money made a huge impact on our lives. Did your parents argue about money often? Or were you the type to have lots of money and can buy anything you want? List down all the words you can associate with money. This will help you realize whether you see money as a positive aspect of human life or otherwise. When you start to think of money as a useful and beneficial tool which can be used in a constructive way, you will definitely attract wealth and financial abundance.

Chapter 11: Reasons why the Law of Attraction isn't Working for you

The Law of attraction states that we attract what we think about. If you always think positively, positive things will come to you. If you always worry and think of negative things, then, negative things will happen to you. A lot of people believe that there are really a lot of benefits to being positive but there are times when the law of attraction just doesn't seem to work at all. Sometimes, no matter how we hard force ourselves to think about money and getting money, we still come back home empty-handed at the end of the day.

It was already said that negative thoughts and beliefs produce money blocks but what could be some of the reasons why the law of attraction does not work in favor of us?

Let's take a look at these reasons...We might be guilty of some unknowingly.

1. Doubts:
Look inside yourself and be honest. You may be harboring some doubts deep inside you and when you start to doubt the effectiveness or the truth behind the law of attraction; it will not work totally for you. It will only work fully if you believe it wholeheartedly.

2. Saying one thing and performing the opposite:

This is still a reflection of doubt towards the law of attraction. Even if you say you believe it wholeheartedly, if your actions don't clearly show it, the result will still be the same...it will not work for you. When you say you believe, you have to really feel it inside you and your actions should manifest such belief and only then will the law of attraction work in your favor.

3. Dwelling in the past:

Learn to leave the past behind. Everything in the past is over so don't hold yourself back and dwell in the past. Stop blaming yourself for something that has happened. Instead, learn to look forward to the future and believe that your future is bright and full of success. This way, when you believe in the future and leave the negative past behind, positive things will definitely happen to you.

4. Negative thoughts:

The law of attraction is very precise. You attract what you think about and so if your mind is full of negative thoughts, these thoughts become more powerful and instead of positive things happening to you, negative things will come instead...because you attracted them by thinking about them. So stop thinking about negative things. Be positive and the law of attraction will be on your side.

5. Laziness:

Success does not work like magic. You have to work for it. It does not come to you just because you thought about it and believed it while sitting and sleeping throughout your lifetime. Success without hard work is not success at all. If you want to attract the good things that the universe can give you, you have to work hard for it, believe that it will come to you, feel it coming and surely, the law of attraction will grant what you truly desire.

6. Being ungrateful:

When someone gives you something, you have to accept it and appreciate one's generosity by being thankful. Gratefulness will make the other person want to give you more in the future. But if you don't show gratitude, no one will be happy to give to you. Check yourself and ask, "Am I being ungrateful"? If you are, then it's about time for you to change that attitude and thank the universe for giving you something you are happy about.

7. Feeling of being unworthy:

Another reason why the law of attraction is not working for you is because you might be thinking that you are unworthy of such a blessing. If you want to win the lottery for example, you have to believe and really feel that you deserve to win. Otherwise it will not be given to you.

Chapter 12: How can EFT Raise your Vibration?

How can EFT raise our vibrations?

In every EFT session, the first thing that we will be asked to do is to think of some problems or issues and then tap on some specific points on our body. By tapping on these points, the physical level changes which in turn also affects and changes our emotional state.

EFT applies the principle that whatever we think about or whatever we vibrate (things not being said) will reach the universe by means of communicating our energetic posture or position.

The vibrations that we emit will be heard by the Universe and in turn it will return to us similar experiences for more vibration and feelings similar to what we have initially emitted.

The Universe can never be fooled by pretending to be joyful when we are not deep down inside. This is because the Universe does not read what we say and do but our vibrations.

This is where EFT comes into the picture. EFT can greatly help in releasing negative energies and conflict in our system so we can vibrate more uplifting and positive space.

When the Universe felt the positive vibration coming from us, it will send back positive signals that will affect us positively as well. The Law of attraction will grant us what we have been asking for.

√ Here are the important things to be considered with EFT tapping:

a. Choose a <u>specific</u> problem

b. Believe and accept that you completely and deeply love yourself no matter what circumstances you are in.

c. Tap on the points within your energy system to help you relieve tension and stress as well as conflicts that have been stored within your system.

This is the perfect way to raise your vibration through EFT tapping in accordance with the Law of attraction.

EFT and the Law of Attraction

You probably have heard and learned so much about the law of attraction. As you know, when you don't seem to be getting what you want, that means there is some resistance...so what could this resistance be? It may be a limiting belief, a doubt or the improper way of life which clearly contradict what you really desire.

This resistance or limiting blocks must be removed or cleared in order for your desires to truly manifest and vibrate to the Universe.

There's no better way to effectively and efficiently remove these limiting blocks except through EFT (Emotional Freedom Technique) tapping. This method can remove even the deep-seated blocks found in the subconscious.

EFT is one of the best and most powerful body and mind techniques that are effective for clearing emotional blocks that hinder us from manifesting and vibrating what we truly desire. People can't seem to believe it at first but the method of tapping on particular acupuncture points on the skin while simultaneously expressing one's emotions and feelings about something can truly open the door for him to get what he really desires deep down inside.

The results are fast and immediate so the clients can tell whether it is effective or not. Tapping these acupuncture points provide access to the subconscious mind and can remove the resistance blocks and when these blocks have been fully removed through EFT tapping, the Law of Attraction can then work completely for you.

Key points to make EFT and Law of Attraction work

Here are some key points to make EFT and Law of Attraction work in conjunction with each other:

The law of attraction is always working 24 hours a day nonstop

The Universe doesn't hear what you say and do but your vibrations which are things that are unsaid but manifested in the subconscious.

Knowledge of the Law of attraction benefits the person as it provides more power in one's life thereby making a person feel less like a victim but a controller of his own life.

Vibrations can be controlled if we know how to make sound choices and focus on changing negative thoughts and actions into positive ones.

To change your vibration, EFT is the fastest and most effective method to be employed.

Now, here is an important question that you might want to ask: Since EFT makes us focus on the negative things (remember that at the start of the EFT session, you will be asked to think about the negative issues or problems you are having) **will this very act of thinking on the negative issues and problems make us attract more negative elements** (law of attraction is applied) **and make things worse for us?**

Fortunately, there is no negative effect on the person even if he is made to think about his own problems and issues through EFT. The law of attraction really attracts what we think about but the EFT method only lets us think of negative things to access them from our subconscious and clear them away for a much more positive and uplifting vibration.

This means that we need to stop resisting what we truly feel. Through EFT, our deepest feelings will float to the surface and will eventually be released into thin air. After this step, you already reached the vibrational position to allow positive energies enter your system and get what you want.

With the use of EFT, we can target a particular emotion which can sometimes be referred to by experts and practitioners as the 'truth' and we can affirm if these feelings are responsible for our negative vibrations. EFT reveals the truth and lets us recognize it by bringing it in front of our eyes to pinpoint. That is why it is important to be specific during the EFT session.

Instead of saying "I hate her", say why you hate her. "I hate her because she did this and that and it hurt me". When you say things like this, you are closer to the truth and it will be easier for you to let go and clear this negative feeling if you know what it is and what caused it. EFT is indeed the fastest and most effective method to relieve negative emotions and replace them with positive ones. It may not be able to change what happened so the event may remain the same, but EFT changes the experience, the memory, the emotions and perception about the events that happened. Only when we are truly relieved of these negative feelings and energies, can the Law of Attraction truly penetrate and work fully in our system and give us what we want.

EFT does not tolerate pretensions. The Law of Attraction will not work for you if you are just pretending. For example, pretending you don't hate your boss at work cannot guarantee that you are not emitting negative vibrations and energies towards the Universe. You know how transparent humans can be. Our real feelings still show no matter how hard we try to hide it.

EFT is all about relief. When we have been finally relieved of the negative things we are storing deep inside us, we invite the things we truly desire through numerous channels and the Universe will be able to hear our positive vibrations and as a result, we attract the things that we want and get it.

The manifestations of this positive aura vibrate in a better place. Then things will start to be on a better light as well...relationships, money, coincidences, career opportunities, love, guidance, peace and serendipity.

If you want to be rich but you are worried about your job or the expenses you have to shoulder at home, don't pretend that you are not affected. Acknowledge it and release the worries. Think of the future and believe that you will be able to excel in your job and will be promoted and eventually you will start to earn more and more and get what you want.

Chapter 13: The Basic Recipe for Attracting Money & Financial Wealth

√ **The Basic Recipe for Attracting Money & Financial Wealth**

The basic EFT "recipe" consists of the following four steps, which will be discussed in detail in the next chapters:

Step 0 - Drink water

Step 1 - Tune in and rate

Close your eyes. Take a deep breath as you inspect your whole body for any tightness or physical pain. On a scale of zero to ten (zero being "no pain" and ten being "worst pain"), how will I rate my pain?

The answer to this question will be the rating that you will use as a baseline. Keep in mind that the more detail you have about your pain, the higher your chances of making EFT work for you.

Step 2 – Clearing of psychological reversal

Psychologically reversed is a condition wherein the energetic field that surrounds the specific area where the issue occurs is reversed.

This is the reason why this step is very important. However, clearing your psychological reversal is quite simple to accomplish – and it doesn't come with any negative effect.

To perform psychological reversal for wealth and money issues, tap the "karate point". You may choose the hand, which feels more comfortable for you. Use the four fingers of your dominant hand to tap on the dotted area of the other hand. Tap about 7 seconds for each statement. Continue tapping until you have finished saying all the following statements:

- **Although I am not attracting money and financial wealth, I still love and fully accept myself.**

- **Although I am not attracting money and financial wealth, I forgive myself for whatever I have done to contribute to the pain.**

- **Although I am not attracting money and financial wealth, I forgive the other people who have added to my pain**

- **Although I am not attracting money and financial wealth, I will forever love and fully accept myself.**

Repeat psychological reversal three times. Make sure that you say the statements aloud and energetically, as if what the statements mean are actually true even though you do not fully believe them. I know it may sometimes be difficult to say something that you do not truly believe in. However, just **trust in the process** and you will eventually feel in your heart that you are starting to believe those statements. However, you can say the statements silently or by heart as you breathe.

Step 3 – Tap

Here are the steps in tapping. Tap about 7 seconds on each of the points.

1. Tap on the first point while saying the four statements. Continue tapping until you have said all statements.

2. Go to and tap the second point while saying the four statements.

3. Repeat the tapping and the statements until you have completed all eight points.

4. After you have finished, inhale and exhale deeply.

5. Drink just enough water.

Start tapping your index and middle fingers on the tapping points of your body:

Eyebrow point, which is located closest to the inside end of your left eyebrow. Do make sure though, that you do not go down to your nose's bridge.

"Although I am not attracting money
and financial wealth, I still love and fully
accept myself."

"Although I am not attracting money
and financial wealth, I forgive myself for whatever
I have done to contribute to the pain."

"Although I am not attracting money
and financial wealth, I forgive the other
people who have added to my pain."

"Although I am not attracting money
and financial wealth, I will forever love
and fully accept myself."

<u>Side-of-the-eye point</u>, which is located closest to the outside end of your right eye. Make sure that you do not poke your eyeball. If you suddenly notice that your vision started to become blurred or you see a flash of light or darkness, it means that the incorrect spot is being tapped.

"Although I am not attracting money
and financial wealth, I still love and
fully accept myself."

"Although I am not attracting money
and financial wealth, I forgive myself for
whatever I have done to contribute to the pain."

"Although I am not attracting money
and financial wealth, I forgive the other
people who have added to my pain"

"Although I am not attracting money
and financial wealth, I will forever love
and fully accept myself."

Under-the-eye point, which is located on your left cheekbone just under your pupil. If you have sinusitis, you can choose to tap very lightly.

"Although I am not attracting money
and financial wealth, I still love and fully
accept myself."

"Although I am not attracting money
and financial wealth, I forgive myself for
whatever I have done to contribute to the pain."

"Although I am not attracting money
and financial wealth, I forgive the other people
who have added to my pain."

"Although I am not attracting money
and financial wealth, I will forever love and fully
accept myself."

Under-the-nose point, which is located exactly between your nose and your upper lip.

"Although I am not attracting money
and financial wealth, I still love and fully
accept myself."

"Although I am not attracting money
and financial wealth, I forgive myself for
whatever I have done to contribute to the pain."

"Although I am not attracting money
and financial wealth, I forgive the other people
who have added to my pain."

"Although I am not attracting money
and financial wealth, I will forever love
and fully accept myself."

<u>Under-the-mouth point</u>, which is located on the dip that connects your chin and lower lip.

"Although I am not attracting money
and financial wealth, I still love and fully
accept myself."

"Although I am not attracting money
and financial wealth, I forgive myself for
whatever I have done to contribute to the pain."

"Although I am not attracting money
and financial wealth, I forgive the other people
who have added to my pain."

"Although I am not attracting money
and financial wealth, I will forever love and
fully accept myself."

Collarbone point, which is located exactly where your collarbone and your sternum meet.

"Although I am not attracting money and financial wealth, I still love and fully accept myself."

"Although I am not attracting money and financial wealth, I forgive myself for whatever I have done to contribute to the pain."

"Although I am not attracting money and financial wealth, I forgive the other people who have added to my pain."

"Although I am not attracting money and financial wealth, I will forever love and fully accept myself."

Under-the-arm point, which is located on the side of your body that is nearer the back side than the front – around four inches down your armpit. If you poke your fingers in the area, you will find it as the tenderest part. To be that you are tapping on the right spot, use all your four fingers when you tap on the under-the-arm point.

"Although I am not attracting money and financial wealth, I still love and fully accept myself."

"Although I am not attracting money
and financial wealth, I forgive myself for
whatever I have done to contribute to the pain."

"Although I am not attracting money
and financial wealth, I forgive the other
people who have added to my pain."

"Although I am not attracting money
and financial wealth, I will forever love
and fully accept myself."

Top-of-the-head point, which is the peak or highest point on the top of your head.

"Although I am not attracting money
and financial wealth, I still love and
fully accept myself."

"Although I am not attracting money
and financial wealth, I forgive myself for
whatever I have done to contribute to the pain."

"Although I am not attracting money
and financial wealth, I forgive the other people
who have added to my pain."

"Although I am not attracting money
and financial wealth, I will forever love
and fully accept myself."

Step 4 – Tune in and re-rate

Inhale and exhale deeply. Also, take another sip of water. When you are ready, tune in to the point of emotional pain again and ask the following questions:

- Did the intensity of the pain decrease, increase, or stay the same?

- Did any image, vision, or thought entered your mind while you were tapping the different body points?

- Were there any memory or person you remembered?

If you answered "yes" to any of these questions, whatever entered your mind might be connected to the pain that you are currently working on.

Rate how you feel now using the same scale of zero to ten.

Chapter 14: Advanced EFT Tapping Scripts - Cleaning Negative Beliefs about Money

It is important to realize by this time that money is an important energy in this world that is found anywhere and is abundant if we know how to attract it to us. Our belief that money is limited and is hard to earn is precisely the reason why we stuck in the poor situation we are in right now. Some people believe that money can't grow on trees but the truth is, money can grow if you believe it will grow and if you think money can't give you happiness, it is about time to realize and think that money can give you the freedom to choose the way you want to live your life including your happiness.

So, while the EFT session is ongoing and while tapping on some of your meridian or acupuncture points it is important that you also repeat some scripts of affirmation to make it more effective and soothing for you.

Here are some tapping scripts to help you attract money and financial wealth through EFT.

This chapter provides 3 great detailed scripts for cleaning negative beliefs about money:

Script a - Accept and love the wondrous energy of money

Script b - Believe and feel that you are worthy of money

Script c - Choose to be connected to prosperity infinitely

√ <u>Script a</u> - Accept and Love the Wondrous Energy of Money

<u>Step 0 - Drink water</u>

<u>Step 1 - Tune in and rate</u>

<u>Step 2 – Clearing of psychological reversal</u>

Tap about 7 seconds for each statement on your karate point. Continue tapping until you have finished saying all the following statements:

- Although I am not accepting and love the wondrous energy of money, I still love and fully accept myself.

- Although I am not accepting and love the wondrous energy of money, I forgive myself for whatever I have done to contribute to the pain.

- Although I am not accepting and love the wondrous energy of money, I forgive the other people who have added to my pain

- Although I am not accepting and love the wondrous energy of money, I will forever love and fully accept myself.

Repeat psychological reversal <u>three</u> times.

Step 3 – Tap

Here are the steps in tapping. Repeat tapping about 7 seconds on each of the points.

Start tapping your index and middle fingers on the tapping points of your body:

Eyebrow point
"I accept and love the wondrous energy of money"

Side-of-the-eye point
"I accept and love the wondrous energy of money"

Under-the-eye point
"I accept and love the wondrous energy of money"

Under-the-nose point
"I accept and love the wondrous energy of money"

Under-the-mouth point
"I accept and love the wondrous energy of money"

Collarbone point
"I accept and love the wondrous energy of money"

Under-the-arm point
"I accept and love the wondrous energy of money"

Top-of-the-head point
"I accept and love the wondrous energy of money"

Step 4 – Tune in and re-rate

√ <u>Script b</u> - Believe and feel that you are worthy of money

<u>Step 0 - Drink water</u>

<u>Step 1 - Tune in and rate</u>

<u>Step 2 – Clearing of psychological reversal</u>

Tap about 7 seconds for each statement on your karate point. Continue tapping until you have finished saying all the following statements:

- Although I don't believe and feel that I am worthy of money, I still love and fully accept myself.

- Although I don't believe and feel that I am worthy of money, I forgive myself for whatever I have done to contribute to the pain.

- Although I don't believe and feel that I am worthy of money, I forgive the other people who have added to my pain

- Although I don't believe and feel that I am worthy of money, I will forever love and fully accept myself.

Repeat psychological reversal <u>three</u> times.

Step 3 – Tap

Here are the steps in tapping. Repeat tapping about 7 seconds on each of the points.

Start tapping your index and middle fingers on the tapping points of your body:

Eyebrow point
"I believe and feel that I am worthy of money"

Side-of-the-eye point
"I believe and feel that I am worthy of money"

Under-the-eye point
"I believe and feel that I am worthy of money"

Under-the-nose point
"I believe and feel that I am worthy of money"

Under-the-mouth point
"I believe and feel that I am worthy of money"

Collarbone point
"I believe and feel that I am worthy of money"

Under-the-arm point
"I believe and feel that I am worthy of money"

Top-of-the-head point
"I believe and feel that I am worthy of money"

<u>Step 4 – Tune in and re-rate</u>

√ <u>Script c</u> - Choose to be connected to prosperity infinitely

<u>Step 0 - Drink water</u>

<u>Step 1 - Tune in and rate</u>

<u>Step 2 – Clearing of psychological reversal</u>

Tap about 7 seconds for each statement on your karate point. Continue tapping until you have finished saying all the following statements:

- Although I don't choose to be connected to prosperity infinitely, I still love and fully accept myself.

- Although I don't choose to be connected to prosperity infinitely, I forgive myself for whatever I have done to contribute to the pain.

- Although I don't choose to be connected to prosperity infinitely, I forgive the other people who have added to my pain

- Although I don't choose to be connected to prosperity infinitely, I will forever love and fully accept myself.

Repeat psychological reversal <u>three</u> times.

Step 3 – Tap

Here are the steps in tapping. Repeat tapping about 7 seconds on each of the points.

Start tapping your index and middle fingers on the tapping points of your body:

Eyebrow point
"I choose to be connected to prosperity infinitely"

Side-of-the-eye point
"I choose to be connected to prosperity infinitely"

Under-the-eye point
"I choose to be connected to prosperity infinitely"

Under-the-nose point
"I choose to be connected to prosperity infinitely"

Under-the-mouth point
"I choose to be connected to prosperity infinitely"

Collarbone point
"I choose to be connected to prosperity infinitely"

Under-the-arm point
"I choose to be connected to prosperity infinitely"

Top-of-the-head point
"I choose to be connected to prosperity infinitely"

Step 4 – Tune in and re-rate

Chapter 15: Advanced EFT Tapping Scripts- Producing your Positive "Wealth Frequency" that Transforms your Relationships to Money

This chapter provides 3 great detailed scripts for producing your positive "wealth frequency" that transforms your relationships to money:

<u>Script a</u> - Let go of all the reasons why you can't be prosperous
<u>Script b</u> - Feel rich despite what your bank account tells you
<u>Script c</u> - See and feel abundance all around you

√ <u>Script a</u> - Let go of all the reasons why you can't be prosperous

<u>Step 0 - Drink water</u>

<u>Step 1 - Tune in and rate</u>

Step 2 – Clearing of psychological reversal

Tap about 7 seconds for each statement on your karate point. Continue tapping until you have finished saying all the following statements:

- Although I don't let go of all the reasons why I can't be prosperous, I still love and fully accept myself.

- Although I don't let go of all the reasons why I can't be prosperous, I forgive myself for whatever I have done to contribute to the pain.

- Although I don't let go of all the reasons why I can't be prosperous, I forgive the other people who have added to my pain

- Although I don't let go of all the reasons why I can't be prosperous, I will forever love and fully accept myself.

Repeat psychological reversal <u>three</u> times.

Step 3 – Tap

Here are the steps in tapping. Repeat tapping about 7 seconds on each of the points.

Start tapping your index and middle fingers on the tapping points of your body:

Eyebrow point
"I let go of all the reasons why I can't be prosperous"

Side-of-the-eye point
"I let go of all the reasons why I can't be prosperous"

Under-the-eye point
"I let go of all the reasons why I can't be prosperous"

Under-the-nose point
"I let go of all the reasons why I can't be prosperous"

Under-the-mouth point
"I let go of all the reasons why I can't be prosperous"

Collarbone point
"I let go of all the reasons why I can't be prosperous"

Under-the-arm point
"I let go of all the reasons why I can't be prosperous"

Top-of-the-head point
"I let go of all the reasons why I can't be prosperous"

Step 4 – Tune in and re-rate

√ Script b - Feel rich despite what your bank account tells you

Step 0 - Drink water

Step 1 - Tune in and rate

Step 2 – Clearing of psychological reversal

Tap about 7 seconds for each statement on your karate point. Continue tapping until you have finished saying all the following statements:

- Although I don't feel rich despite what my bank account tells me, I still love and fully accept myself.

- Although I don't feel rich despite what my bank account tells me, I forgive myself for whatever I have done to contribute to the pain.

- Although I don't feel rich despite what my bank account tells me, I forgive the other people who have added to my pain

- Although I don't feel rich despite what my bank account tells me, I will forever love and fully accept myself.

Repeat psychological reversal three times.

Step 3 – Tap

Here are the steps in tapping. Repeat tapping about 7 seconds on each of the points.

Start tapping your index and middle fingers on the tapping points of your body:

Eyebrow point
"I feel rich despite what my bank account tells me"

Side-of-the-eye point
"I feel rich despite what my bank account tells me"

Under-the-eye point
"I feel rich despite what my bank account tells me"

Under-the-nose point
"I feel rich despite what my bank account tells me"

Under-the-mouth point
"I feel rich despite what my bank account tells me"

Collarbone point
"I feel rich despite what my bank account tells me"

Under-the-arm point
"I feel rich despite what my bank account tells me"

Top-of-the-head point
"I feel rich despite what my bank account tells me"

Step 4 – Tune in and re-rate

√ <u>Script c</u> - See and Feel Abundance all around you

<u>Step 0 - Drink water</u>

<u>Step 1 - Tune in and rate</u>

<u>Step 2 – Clearing of psychological reversal</u>

Tap about 7 seconds for each statement on your karate point. Continue tapping until you have finished saying all the following statements:

- **Although I can't see and feel abundance all around me, I still love and fully accept myself.**

- **Although I can't see and feel abundance all around me, I forgive myself for whatever I have done to contribute to the pain.**

- **Although I can't see and feel abundance all around me, I forgive the other people who have added to my pain**

- **Although I can't see and feel abundance all around me, I will forever love and fully accept myself.**

Repeat psychological reversal <u>three</u> times.

Step 3 – Tap

Here are the steps in tapping. Repeat tapping about 7 seconds on each of the points.

Start tapping your index and middle fingers on the tapping points of your body:

Eyebrow point
"I can see and feel abundance all around me"

Side-of-the-eye point
"I can see and feel abundance all around me"

Under-the-eye point
"I can see and feel abundance all around me"

Under-the-nose point
"I can see and feel abundance all around me"

Under-the-mouth point
"I can see and feel abundance all around me"

Collarbone point
"I can see and feel abundance all around me"

Under-the-arm point
"I can see and feel abundance all around me"

Top-of-the-head point
"I can see and feel abundance all around me"

Step 4 – Tune in and re-rate

Chapter 16: Advanced EFT Tapping Scripts - Manifesting and Attracting Wealth and Financial Abundance

This chapter provides three great detailed scripts for manifesting and attracting wealth and financial abundance:

<u>Script a</u> - Always have more than enough money for your needs

<u>Script b</u> - Believe and feel that you have everything in order to be successful

<u>Script c</u> - Letting your life become easier and prosperous now

Script a
Always have more than enough money for your needs

Step 0 - Drink water

Step 1 - Tune in and rate

Step 2 – Clearing of psychological reversal

Tap about 7 seconds for each statement on your karate point. Continue tapping until you have finished saying all the following statements:

- Although I don't always have more than enough money for my needs, I still love and fully accept myself.

- Although I don't always have more than enough money for my needs, I forgive myself for whatever I have done to contribute to the pain.

- Although I don't always have more than enough money for my needs, I forgive the other people who have added to my pain

- Although I don't always have more than enough money for my needs, I will forever love and fully accept myself.

Repeat psychological reversal <u>three</u> times.

Step 3 – Tap

Here are the steps in tapping. Repeat tapping about 7 seconds on each of the points.

Start tapping your index and middle fingers on the tapping points of your body:

Eyebrow point
"I always have more than enough money for my needs"

Side-of-the-eye point
"I always have more than enough money for my needs"

Under-the-eye point
"I always have more than enough money for my needs"

Under-the-nose point
"I always have more than enough money for my needs"

Under-the-mouth point
"I always have more than enough money for my needs"

Collarbone point
"I always have more than enough money for my needs"

Under-the-arm point
"I always have more than enough money for my needs"

Top-of-the-head point
"I always have more than enough money for my needs"

Step 4 – Tune in and re-rate

Script b - Believe and feel that you have everything in order to be successful

Step 0 - Drink water

Step 1 - Tune in and rate

Step 2 – Clearing of psychological reversal

Tap about 7 seconds for each statement on your karate point. Continue tapping until you have finished saying all the following statements:

- Although I don't believe and feel that I have everything in order to be successful, I still love and fully accept myself.

- Although I don't believe and feel that I have everything in order to be successful, I forgive myself for whatever I have done to contribute to the pain.

- Although don't believe and feel that I have everything in order to be successful, I forgive the other people who have added to my pain

- Although I don't believe and feel that I have everything in order to be successful, I will forever love and fully accept myself.

Repeat psychological reversal three times.

Step 3 – Tap

Here are the steps in tapping. Repeat tapping about 7 seconds on each of the points.

Start tapping your index and middle fingers on the tapping points of your body:

Eyebrow point
 "I believe and I feel that I have everything in order to be successful"

Side-of-the-eye point
"I believe and I feel that I have everything in order to be successful"

Under-the-eye point
"I believe and I feel that I have everything in order to be successful"

Under-the-nose point
"I believe and I feel that I have everything in order to be successful"

Under-the-mouth point
"I believe and I feel that I have everything in order to be successful"

Collarbone point
"I believe and I feel that I have everything in order to be successful"

Under-the-arm point
"I believe and I feel that I have everything in order to be successful"

Top-of-the-head point
"I believe and I feel that I have everything in order to be successful"

Step 4 – Tune in and re-rate

Script c - Letting your life become easier and prosperous now

Step 0 - Drink water

Step 1 - Tune in and rate

Step 2 – Clearing of psychological reversal

Tap about 7 seconds for each statement on your karate point. Continue tapping until you have finished saying all the following statements:

- Although I am not letting my life become easier and prosperous now, I still love and fully accept myself.

- Although I am not letting my life become easier and prosperous now, I forgive myself for whatever I have done to contribute to the pain.

- Although I am not letting my life become easier and prosperous now, I forgive the other people who have added to my pain

- Although I am not letting my life become easier and prosperous now, I will forever love and fully accept myself.

Repeat psychological reversal three times.

Step 3 – Tap

Here are the steps in tapping. Repeat tapping about 7 seconds on each of the points.

Start tapping your index and middle fingers on the tapping points of your body:

Eyebrow point
"I am letting my life become easier and prosperous now"

Side-of-the-eye point
"I am letting my life become easier and prosperous now"

Under-the-eye point
"I am letting my life become easier and prosperous now"

Under-the-nose point
"I am letting my life become easier and prosperous now"

Under-the-mouth point
"I am letting my life become easier and prosperous now"

Collarbone point
"I am letting my life become easier and prosperous now"

Under-the-arm point
"I am letting my life become easier and prosperous now"

Top-of-the-head point
"I am letting my life become easier and prosperous now"

Step 4 – Tune in and re-rate

Part 4
Tapping for Improving Relationships

Manifesting and Attracting
Romantic Relationship You Desire

Chapter 17: Improving Relationships

You can use EFT to improve your personal relationships. Many studies have demonstrated that EFT improves people's moods and ways of thinking. These two factors translate to better relationships because internal states affect how a person behaves and relates to others.

Here's a quick guide on how you can use EFT to increase your social interactions and resolve your relationship issues.

The EFT Method

Improving relationships via EFT involves the following:

Determining exactly what you want to get or get rid of. The goal of EFT as a curative and life-enhancing therapy is to give you what you want and need. If you're interested in enhancing your relationships, think about where you're having problems and how you would like to be relationship-wise. Try your best to give details – doing so is therapeutic in itself since it brings your focus and control to what normally lies beyond your awareness. Also, your problem-solving and idea-generating mind will have material to work on once you pinpoint things that are important to you.

Phrasing your intention in a way that your mind can easily process it. Your conscious will is a small part of your entire mind, and these other mental components may misunderstand your intentions if you're unclear about them.

Consider these phrases or 'scripts' as instructions for your deeper mind and clarify your scripts.

Relaxing and deep breathing to put you into a receptive state. To access the programmable state of mind, you need to put your defensive and easily distracted mind at ease.

Observing your internal state. This gives you a sense of where you are and how the methods are affecting you. Rate the intensity of your emotions and record them.

Tapping the appropriate locations in the body. This activates the energy channels that are the focal points of EFT energy manipulation.

Stating the intentions while tapping. This imprints your intentions to your energy while embedding them to your subconscious. Thus, you reprogram yourself psychologically and energetically.

Paying attention to internal changes. This will tell you whether to continue or stop. Repeat the process until you feel that it's enough.

√ Script Making for Relationships

Scripts must be specific, simple, and honest. They can be rants, goals, or a combination of both. EFT scripts differ from certain practices because they encourage the verbalization of negative emotions in order for them to be released. Feel free to speak your hurts out loud; don't worry that they will attract negative situations to you. Instead, think about it as your way of purging your energy system of unwanted blockages so that your vital forces can run smoothly again. Don't forget to include your desires to redirect your energy to desirable paths.

Include the names of the people you want to deal with, may they be your friends, your family, or your partner/s. While saying the script, imagine them. Speaking the names loudly or in your head and visualizing their images strengthen your connection with them.

You can have short scripts, long scripts, dramatic laments or straightforward quips. Whatever your style may be, keep your goals in mind and feel passionate about getting the relationships you truly want.

√ Relationship-Specific Issues

Find an issue you'd like to work with. Here are some ideas to jog your thoughts:

Confidence. Being confident is feeling empowered to do something while overcoming hesitation and fear. Be clear about where you want confidence in so that your mind will have an easier time responding to your request. Do you want to be charismatic so potential mates gravitate to you? Gathering courage to speak your mind about an issue with your significant other? Turn this into a phrase such as, "I find the strength to talk with _ about _." Or, "Even though I feel anxious whenever I meet _, I accept my insecurities and I will become comfortable with myself."

Communication. Energy blockages are related to communication troubles. It goes both ways: if you have problems with your energy, you might find it difficult to express yourself freely, or if your expression is constantly hampered, you might develop energetic imbalances. Do the EFT tapping methods to clear your channels. State affirmations: "I am a great communicator," or "I accept my fear of talking and I will find inner peace."

Finding a Partner. Relationships are energetic exchanges; when you fix your energetic problems, it's likely that your relationships will also fall into alignment. Loosen up your energy and vocalize statements like, "I love myself and I am attracting a loving partner to my life."

Moving On. Resentment, guilt, jealousy, and a host of other negative emotions can hold you back from experiencing rewarding connections with others. Feel the pain, acknowledge it, while expressing your intent to leave it behind you. "I am hurt, but I choose to move on and find better things in life."

EFT has endless applications for your relationships. The trick is to increase yourself awareness and listen to your heart's desires. Bring both dreams and distress to the surface, tap away, and anticipate positive changes in yourself and your life.

√ Scripts for manifesting and attracting romantic relationship you desire

<u>Step 0 - Drink water</u>

<u>Step 1 - Tune in and rate</u>

<u>Step 2 – Clearing of psychological reversal</u>

Tap about 7 seconds for each statement on your karate point. Continue tapping until you have finished saying all the following statements:

<u>Step 3 – Tap</u>

Here are the steps in tapping. There are three rounds. In each round repeat tapping about 7 seconds on each of the points. Start tapping your index and middle fingers on the tapping points of your body.

<u>Step 4 – Tune in and re-rate</u>

√ <u>Script 1</u> - Fears about starting a relationship

<u>Clearing of psychological reversal</u>

Tap about 7 seconds for each statement on your karate point. Continue tapping until you have finished saying all the following statements (Repeat psychological reversal three times):

- Although I have fears about starting a relationship, I still love and fully accept myself.

- Although I don't always attract my ideal soul-mate, I forgive myself for whatever I have done to contribute to the emotional pain.

- Although I fear of intimacy, I forgive the other people who have added to my fear.

- Although my partner might reject me, I will forever love and fully accept myself.

Here are the steps in tapping. Repeat tapping about 7 seconds on each of the points.

Start tapping your index and middle fingers on the tapping points of your body. (rounds 1-3).

Round 1 – Tap

<u>Eyebrow point</u>
"Fears about starting a relationship"

<u>Side-of-the-eye point</u>
"Fears about starting a relationship"

<u>Under-the-eye point</u>
"Don't always attract my ideal soul-mate"

<u>Under-the-nose point</u>
"Don't always attract my ideal soul-mate"

<u>Under-the-mouth point</u>
"Fear of intimacy"

<u>Collarbone point</u>
"Fear of intimacy"

<u>Under-the-arm point</u>
"My partner might reject me"

<u>Top-of-the-head point</u>
"My partner might reject me"

Round 2 – Tap

Eyebrow point
"I am reducing my fears about starting a relationship"

Side-of-the-eye point
"I am reducing my fears about starting a relationship"

Under-the-eye point
"I sometimes attract my ideal soul-mate"

Under-the-nose point
"I sometimes attract my ideal soul-mate"

Under-the-mouth point
"I am reducing my fear of intimacy"

Collarbone point
"I am reducing my fear of intimacy"

Under-the-arm point
"My partner might accept me"

Top-of-the-head point
"My partner might accept me"

Round 3 – Tap

Eyebrow point
"I can release my fears about starting a relationship"

Side-of-the-eye point
"I am releasing my fears about starting a relationship"

Under-the-eye point
"I can attract my ideal soul-mate"

Under-the-nose point
"I am attracting my ideal soul-mate"

Under-the-mouth point
"I am reducing my fear of intimacy"

Collarbone point
"I am releasing my fear of intimacy"

Under-the-arm point
"My partner can accept me"

Top-of-the-head point
"My partner is going to accept me"

√ **Script 2 - Unhealthy Relationships**

Clearing of psychological reversal

Tap about 7 seconds for each statement on your karate point. Continue tapping until you have finished saying all the following statements. Repeat psychological reversal <u>three</u> times:

- **Although I had unhealthy relationships,
  I still love and fully accept myself.**

- **Although I don't attract the romantic relationship I desire,
  I forgive myself for whatever I have done to contribute to the emotional pain.**

- **Although my relationships make me feel frustrated,
  I forgive my partners who have added to my frustration.**

- **Although I am in a relationship that makes me feel bad,
  I will forever love and fully accept myself.**

Here are the steps in tapping. Repeat tapping about 7 seconds on each of the points.

Start tapping your index and middle fingers on the tapping points of your body (rounds 1-3).

Round 1 – Tap

Eyebrow point
"Unhealthy relationships"

Side-of-the-eye point
"Bad relationships"

Under-the-eye point
"Don't attract the romantic relationship I desire"

Under-the-nose point
"Ever attracted the romantic relationship I desired"

Under-the-mouth point
"Feel frustration"

Collarbone point
"Feel anger"

Under-the-arm point
"Feel bad"

Top-of-the-head point
"Feel fear"

Round 2 – Tap

Eyebrow point
"I can reduce my fears about unhealthy relationships"

Side-of-the-eye point
"I can reduce my fears about bad a relationships"

Under-the-eye point
"I sometimes attract the romantic relationship I desire"

Under-the-nose point
"I sometimes attract my ideal relationship I desire"

Under-the-mouth point
"I can reduce my frustration"

Collarbone point
"I can reduce my anger"

Under-the-arm point
"My relationships make me feel less frustrated"

Top-of-the-head point
"My bad relationships make me feel less frustrated"

Round 3 – Tap

Eyebrow point
"I can release my fears about unhealthy relationships"

Side-of-the-eye point
"I am releasing my fears about unhealthy relationships"

Under-the-eye point
"I can attract the romantic relationship I desire"

Under-the-nose point
"I am attracting the romantic relationship I desire"

Under-the-mouth point
"I am reducing my frustration"

Collarbone point
"I am releasing my anger"

Under-the-arm point
"My relationships make me feel good"

Top-of-the-head point
"My relationships are going to be great"

√ **Script 3 - Expecting to be Rejected**

Clearing of psychological reversal

Tap about 7 seconds for each statement on your karate point. Continue tapping until you have finished saying all the following statements. Repeat psychological reversal three times:

- **Although I am expecting to be rejected, I still love and fully accept myself.**

- **Although I have fears of the unknown, I forgive myself for whatever I have done to contribute to the emotional pain.**

- **Although my fear of being hurt emotionally, I forgive my partners who have added to my frustration.**

- **Although I had too many bad dates, I will forever love and fully accept myself.**

Here are the steps in tapping. Repeat tapping about 7 seconds on each of the points.

Start tapping your index and middle fingers on the tapping points of your body. (rounds 1-3).

Round 1 – Tap

Eyebrow point
"To be rejected"

Side-of-the-eye point
"To be rejected"

Under-the-eye point
"Fears of the unknown"

Under-the-nose point
"Fears of new relationship"

Under-the-mouth point
"Fear of being hurt"

Collarbone point
"Being hurt emotionally"

Under-the-arm point
"Too many bad dates"

Top-of-the-head point
"Bad dates"

Round 2 – Tap

<u>Eyebrow point</u>
"I can reduce my fears to be rejected"

<u>Side-of-the-eye point</u>
"I sometimes reduce my fears to be rejected"

<u>Under-the-eye point</u>
"I can trust in another person"

<u>Under-the-nose point</u>
"I sometimes trust in another person"

<u>Under-the-mouth point</u>
"I can open myself to someone new"

<u>Collarbone point</u>
"I can reduce my fear to someone new"

<u>Under-the-arm point</u>
"I can reduce my fears of the unknown"

<u>Top-of-the-head point</u>
"I sometimes reduce my fears of the unknown"

Round 3 – Tap

Eyebrow point
"I can release my fears of the unknown"

Side-of-the-eye point
"I can overcome my fears of the unknown"

Under-the-eye point
"I will be excited to try new things"

Under-the-nose point
"I can love to try new things"

Under-the-mouth point
"I can overcome the fear of being hurt emotionally"

Collarbone point
"I want to find a loving partner"

Under-the-arm point
"I can enjoy dating"

Top-of-the-head point
"My dates are going to be great"

Part 5
Tapping for other common issues

Kids, Sports Performance,
Sleep Problems, Self Confidence

Chapter 18: Tapping for Kids

EFT is a good method that both parents and teachers can use to help children overcome their daily anxieties. Children can easily make use of the tapping technique to soothe any problems that they are encountering in their home or school.

However, there may be some cases where children might find it difficult to deal with their issues due to any lingering negative emotions that they cannot address by themselves. When the children are unable to express their feelings of fear, anger, shame or guilt, even the smallest issues could end up becoming bigger and more complicated in the future.

Therefore, it will be your responsibility as a parent or teacher to help these kids pinpoint the exact issue or emotion that is giving them anxiety. Quickly addressing the issue will prevent the children from negatively acting out on their emotions and causing mayhem at home or at school.

Using EFT in a School Setting

One common problem that children can have in a school setting is being fearful of their teacher. They could be afraid of making a mistake that could cause them to anger their teacher. If left alone, the fear could cause the children to become timid or otherwise more disruptive in class.

Therefore, once a teacher notices any sudden changes in the student's behavior, it is best that they speak with that child instead of using intimidation to establish their control in the classroom. They can ask the student to explain the underlying reason for their fear and give them a corresponding affirmative phrase to combat that anxiety.

One good phrase would be, "Even though the teacher might get mad when I do naughty things, I know that she still cares about me." This phrase will help the student feel more relaxed inside the classroom and help strengthen his relationship with his teacher as well.

Similarly, children could also be experiencing difficulties in dealing with school problems related to their academic performance. Although you might hear them saying that they hate a particular subject, they might simply be feeling frustrated over a difficult new lesson. In such cases you should assist them in discovering the underlying reason for their frustration.

One good starting phrase that you can teach them is, "Even though I am not as good at (supply subject or topic) as the other kids, I am still an awesome kid anyway." Afterwards, you can ask the child other questions that could help you pinpoint the exact cause of his or her anxiety.

He could actually be more worried about displeasing his teacher rather than of being unable to follow the new lesson. In such a case, you can use the phrase "Even though I am worried that the teacher might get mad at me because (supply the learning difficulty), I am still an awesome kid anyway."

Likewise, he might also be feeling anxious about the perception of his peers regarding his performance. Therefore, you can have him recite the phrase, "Even though I get embarrassed when my classmates tease me because (supply specific event), I am still an awesome kid anyway."

Finally, in order to help him feel more confident in his ability, you will have to raise his self-esteem. After all, his negative first impression regarding a specific topic or subject could cause him to shun any related future activities. This means that you will have to teach him a few affirmative statements that will reinforce his belief in his own abilities.

Initially, you can make use of statements such as, "I am smart, I am creative, I am brave, etc." Afterwards, you can help the child create more goal-oriented phrases that will enable them to tackle their specific problems. Phrases such as, "I can learn or pass (supply specific topic), or I will finish all my assignments for today" will help him get into a more successful mindset.

Eventually, after a few rounds of affirmative statements, he will be able feel better about the situation and find renewed motivation to tackle any challenging new subject matter. The teacher will find that his students immediately become more cooperative and enthusiastic in learning new things after they are taught these EFT techniques.

Using EFT at Home

Once the children return from school, it will then be the parent's role to supervise their children's mental and emotional development. Unfortunately, unlike the teachers, parents are not given lunch breaks in between their lessons at home. In fact, parent's often have to be prepared to deal with any anxieties that children might experience from dawn until dusk.

One of the most common problems that many children suffer from is the inability to fall asleep. They might have too many thoughts in their heads that are preventing them from falling asleep. In such cases, you would have to ask them about these thoughts and let them voice out their anxieties. Eventually, once they have shared their issues, you can teach them the phrase, "Even though I have to or want to (supply specific issue), I know that can do them tomorrow when I wake up." In this way they will be able to relax and surrender themselves to sleep.

Another common problem that children experience is suffering from nightmares. Often, these nightmares often cause your children to get scared, worried or even traumatized. As a result, you might want to take these problems onto yourself instead of letting your child suffer.

Nevertheless, it is actually recommended that you let your child learn to self-soothe and tap out these problems on his own. Simply teach him to say the phrase, "Even though my nightmares are scary, I know that they are not real." This phrase will help calm his emotions and allow him to go back to sleep without relying on your assistance.

Ultimately, regardless of the possible issues that may arise, it is best that you only provide the foundation of EFT to your children and allow them to apply the method on their own. After all, they will not always remain under your care.

Childhood is a transitory period that will only last for so long. Therefore, you should allow them to learn and grow as much as they can during that period in their lives. In that way, they will be able to grow into capable adults who can competently make use of EFT to help them achieve emotional growth and progress using their own means.

Chapter 19: Tapping for Enhancing Sports Performance

It is undeniable that being good in sports relies heavily on proper training and physical conditioning. Nevertheless, if you are not mentally strong, you will not be able to attain success in spite of your physical capabilities. Therefore, it is recommended that you also include mental conditioning techniques such as EFT to create a more balanced regimen.

EFT is an easy method that you can use to cause a positive change in your athletic performance. You simply need to think of select affirmative phrases that will engage your mind. Afterwards, you will recite these phrases while stimulating some select acupressure points on your body using tapping motions.

Effects of EFT

Similar to your physical training, you will be able to measure the tangible changes that could result from this mental conditioning technique. Once you consistently apply EFT to your training regimen, you will notice changes not only in your mental strength, but in your physical strength as well.

In fact, one immediate effect of EFT is a noticeable tolerance of physical pain and accelerated recovery from injury. Although, you will not become invincible, you will be less affected and therefore less afraid of getting hurt. As a result, this improvement will give you more confidence to break free from your comfort zones and take more risks.

Likewise, the newfound strength resulting from the training will boost your confidence and help you get over your past performance-related insecurities. In this regard, EFT can be particularly beneficial for athletes who are suffering from any physical issues that are conversely affecting their performance.

Ensuring Sustainability of Performance

Often, the body part that could be causing their pain is also the same body part that is subjected to constant abuse during an athlete's training. Therefore, in such cases, the athlete simply ends up tolerating the pain in order to keep playing the sport that he loves. Unfortunately, that abuse will eventually take its toll on the body part and weaken it to the point of uselessness.

For that reason, it is important to take the time to listen to your body every once in a while. Although, being an athlete does require you to always push yourself beyond your limits, you still have the responsibility to take care of yourself. You should learn to recognize whatever limitations you might have and accept them as part of yourself.

A common EFT technique that you can use in order to enhance your sports performance is to create an affirmative phrase that will target a specific body part. If you are not suffering from any particular physical condition, then that body part could simply be something that you wish to strengthen. In such a case, you could simply be hoping for a more visible result of your training. Therefore, the general phrase you can use is, "Even though I am exhausted from my daily training, I choose to believe that I will succeed due to my efforts."

157

Additionally, you can also use EFT to combat the negative emotions that could stem from your physical insecurities. After all, emotions such as envy, anger, or frustration towards your teammates or partner could only worsen your condition. Therefore, it is best that you address your emotions and say, "Even though I am angry that none of my teammates have to worry about their (supply body part) during our training and tournaments, I choose to be content and happy with myself."

The effect of accepting your emotions instead of keeping them bottled up inside will help free your mind and keep you more focused on your training. Likewise, being more content with your abilities will enable you to better appreciate the things that you are able to accomplish in spite of your shortcomings.

Chapter 20: Tapping for Sleep Problems

Oftentimes, people who suffer from sleep disorders such as insomnia have turned to sleeping pills as a means to help them get a good night's sleep. Unfortunately, these drugs only have a temporary effect. Likewise, overdosing or overdependence on these pills could cause serious repercussions.

Thankfully, these individuals can make use of the EFT technique as a good alternative method to help them safely treat their own sleep disorders over the long term. Additionally, these EFT maneuvers can help them deal not only with the superficial sleep disorder, but also with their more serious underlying causes.

One of the most common EFT techniques that people use to remedy their inability to sleep is to recite a general phrase that can put their mind at ease. Individuals who simply need to calm themselves in order to fall asleep can recite the general affirmation, "Even though I can't fall asleep or I can't seem to quiet my thoughts to get to sleep, I accept myself as I am."

Although this phrase does serve as a good starting point for EFT treatment, it might not always give the desired results. If you feel that there is an actual underlying cause for your insomnia, then it is best that you use a phrase that is more specific to your anxieties. You will have to pinpoint that exact emotional, physical, or psychological problem that causes your sleeplessness so that you can permanently counteract it with the corresponding affirmative phrase.

One of the most common cause of insomnia is feeling overwhelmed with the number of responsibilities that you have to deal with. In that scenario, your guilt in seeking a respite from your responsibilities could be preventing you from falling asleep. Therefore, your affirmation in this case will be, "Even though I have a great responsibility (supply your specific responsibilities), I will be more capable of dealing with these thoughts after I have had a pleasant rest."

Another common cause of sleep deprivation is stress or anxiety. In such cases, you might be feeling afraid of any possible negative outcomes over things that are often out of your control. Therefore, the affirmative phrase you should use should use in this scenario is, "Even though I am worried about (supply your specific anxieties), I choose to remain calm and at peace."

The final common cause of insomnia is anger. In such a case, you will have to pinpoint the direct cause of your resentment and recite, "Even though I am angry or furious with (supply your specific issue), I choose to remain calm." By reciting this phrase, you will be able to quiet your feelings and find your inner peace. Once you are peaceful, you will find it much easier to fall asleep.

Chapter 21: EFT Tapping for Self Confidence

Confidence Builder - Think Positive

Positivity is something every confident person has. Regardless of the situation, truly confident people never lose their poise, even at the face of daunting odds.

People with a positive attitude love who they are and what they do at all times. Positivity adds to one's personality because people are naturally gravitated towards those who present good vibes.

You can enhance your positivity by finding the good in every person or situation, focusing more on the good things and refraining from dishing out unnecessary criticism.

Script 1 - Focusing on the bad things

<u>Clearing of psychological reversal</u>

Tap about 7 seconds for each statement on your karate point.

Continue tapping until you have finished saying all the following statements (Repeat psychological reversal three times):

- **Although I feel focusing more on the bad things, I still love and fully accept that I have these bad things.**

- Although I feel focusing more on the bad things,
  I forgive myself for whatever I have done to contribute
  to the emotional pain.

- Although I feel focusing more on the bad things,
  I forgive the other people who have added to my fear.

Here are the steps in tapping. Repeat tapping about 7 seconds on each of the points. Start tapping your index and middle fingers on the tapping points of your body:

Round 1 – Tap

Eyebrow point
"I feel focusing more on the bad things"

Side-of-the-eye point
"I feel focusing more on the bad things"

Under-the-eye point
"I really feel focusing more on the bad things"

Under-the-nose point
"Sometimes I feel focusing more on the bad things
and it's overwhelming"

Under-the-mouth point
"Sometimes I feel focusing more on the bad things
and it makes me feel out of control"

Collarbone point

"But I can't help but feel focusing more on the bad things"

Under-the-arm point

"I wish I could NOT feel focusing more on the bad things"

Top-of-the-head point

"But I do feel focusing more on the bad things"

Round 2 – Tap

<u>Eyebrow point</u>
"I am focusing on the bad things"

<u>Side-of-the-eye point</u>
"I don't like to focus on the bad things"

<u>Under-the-eye point</u>
"I really feel bad when I am focusing on the bad things"

<u>Under-the-nose point</u>
"Even if I don't like it, I am focusing on the bad things"

<u>Under-the-mouth point</u>
"I wonder what it would be like NOT to feel out of control"

<u>Collarbone point</u>
"But I still feel focusing more on the bad things"

<u>Under-the-arm point</u>
"I wish I could feel better"

<u>Top-of-the-head point</u>
"I can feel differently"

Round 3 – Tap

Eyebrow point
"I still feel focusing more on the bad things"

Side-of-the-eye point
"I still have these bad feelings that I feel when
I'm focusing on the bad things"

Under-the-eye point
"I have my reasons to focus more on the bad things"

Under-the-nose point
"Focusing more on the bad things , holds me back"

Under-the-mouth point
"But I want to learn how to let go"

Collarbone point
"Even if I still focus on the bad things"

Under-the-arm point
"I accept the fact that I bad"

Top-of-the-head point
"But I know can feel much better"

Script 2 – Stop focusing on the bad things

Clearing of psychological reversal

Tap about 7 seconds for each statement on your karate point.

Continue tapping until you have finished saying all the following statements (Repeat psychological reversal three times):

- Although I have felt focusing more on the bad things for so long, I still love and fully accept that I have these bad things.

- Although I had reasons to focus more on the bad things, I forgive myself for whatever I have done to contribute to the emotional pain.

- Although I used to feel focusing more on the bad things, I forgive the other people who have added to my bad feeling.

Round 1 – Tap

Eyebrow point
"Even if I still don't feel better"

Side-of-the-eye point
"And even if I don't focus on the good things"

Under-the-eye point
"I don't have to carry this bad feeling with me"

Under-the-nose point
"I can try stop focusing on the bad things "

Under-the-mouth point
"I want to finally let this bad feeling go"

Collarbone point
"I can have survive without focusing on the bad things"

Under-the-arm point
"I will learn how to let go this bad habit"

Top-of-the-head point
"I accept the fact that sometimes I can feel better"

Round 2 – Tap

Eyebrow point
"Focusing on the bad things is starting to feel less troublesome"

Side-of-the-eye point
"I can choose to let this bad feeling go"

Under-the-eye point
"I am worth the freedom to feel better"

Under-the-nose point
"I can stop focusing more on the bad things"

Under-the-mouth point
"I know this bad feeling used to be important to me"

Collarbone point
"But I choose releasing this bad feeling now"

Under-the-arm point
"I have better things to focus"

Top-of-the-head point
"I can finally stop focusing on the bad things"

Round 3 – Tap

Eyebrow point
"I can stop this bad feeling"

Side-of-the-eye point
"I can choose to let this bad feeling go"

Under-the-eye point
"I choose letting go and thinking positive"

Under-the-nose point
"I choose NOT to feel bad and NOT focusing on the bad things"

Under-the-mouth point
"I can feel better when I am focusing more on the good things"

Collarbone point
"I don't need this bad feeling anymore"

Under-the-arm point
"This bad feeling doesn't control me anymore"

Top-of-the-head point
"I am happy to be free and think positive"

Confidence Builder - Talk with Conviction

One great way to look and feel confident is to sound confident. This is where talking with conviction comes into the picture.

Being a confident talker does not have to mean being more dominant or louder than everyone else. You can show confidence by simply stating what you're going to say with conviction.

To do this, make sure that you speak clearly, at the right tone, and at the right pace. You can start by working on your speaking tone, rhythm, pitch and timing.

Script 3 - Sound unconfident

<u>Clearing of psychological reversal</u>

Tap about 7 seconds for each statement on your karate point.

Continue tapping until you have finished saying all the following statements (Repeat psychological reversal three times):

- **Although I sound unconfident, I still love and fully accept that I have these bad feelings.**

- **Although I still sound unconfident and have remaining painful feelings, I forgive myself for whatever I have done to contribute to the emotional pain.**

- **Although I sound unconfident for so long,
  I forgive the other people who have added
  to my bad feeling.**

Round 1 – Tap

Eyebrow point
"I sound unconfident"

Side-of-the-eye point
"I really sound unconfident"

Under-the-eye point
"Sometimes I sound unconfident"

Under-the-nose point
"Sometimes I sound unconfident and it makes me feel out of control"

Under-the-mouth point
"I do sound unconfident and I can't help it"

Collarbone point
"I sound unconfident even if I don't like it"

Under-the-arm point
"I don't know what it would be like NOT to sound unconfident"

Top-of-the-head point
"I sound unconfident because I still have painful feelings"

Round 2 – Tap

Eyebrow point
"I would really like to sound differently"

Side-of-the-eye point
"I can feel differently when I'm ready"

Under-the-eye point
"I have many reasons to sound unconfident"

Under-the-nose point
"I am willing to let these painful feelings go"

Under-the-mouth point
"I want to learn how to let these painful feelings go"

Collarbone point
"I accept I sound unconfident"

Under-the-arm point
"Even if I still sound unconfident"

Top-of-the-head point
"I still really feel less confident about myself"

Round 3 – Tap

Eyebrow point
"when I sound unconfident, it holds me back"

Side-of-the-eye point
"I deserve to sound confident"

Under-the-eye point
"I have the right to sound confident"

Under-the-nose point
"I can feel better when I am confident"

Under-the-mouth point
"I choose to sound confident forever"

Collarbone point
"I choose to let my bad feelings go"

Under-the-arm point
"I am grateful I can sound confident"

Top-of-the-head point
"I can feel happy when I sound confident"

Confidence Builder - Strike a Balance

Confidence is a character trait that must be balanced to ensure perfect execution. Showing too little confidence would give an image that you're being tentative.

Showing excessive confidence would give an image that you're being arrogant. Both extremes are not conducive to developing self confidence.

This is the reason why you have to strike a balance. Never lose your self-belief, but you don't need to rub it on everyone's faces.

Script 4 - Having unbalanced feeling

<u>Clearing of psychological reversal</u>

Tap about 7 seconds for each statement on your karate point.

Continue tapping until you have finished saying all the following statements (Repeat psychological reversal three times):

- **Although I feel unbalanced,
  I still love and fully accept that I have this bad feeling.**

- **Although I have felt unbalanced for so long,
  I forgive myself for whatever I have done to contribute
  to the emotional pain.**

- Although I still feel unbalanced and I have lots of good reasons to feel unbalanced, I forgive the other people who have added to my bad feeling.

Round 1 – Tap

Eyebrow point
"I feel unbalanced"

Side-of-the-eye point
"I really feel unbalanced and I can't help it"

Under-the-eye point
"Sometimes I feel unbalanced"

Under-the-nose point
"I feel unbalanced and it makes me feel out of control"

Under-the-mouth point
"I wish I could feel balanced but I do feel unbalanced"

Collarbone point
"I feel unbalanced even if I don't like it"

Under-the-arm point
"I have the right to feel unbalanced"

Top-of-the-head point
"But I would really like to feel better"

Round 2 – Tap

Eyebrow point
"I still feel unbalanced, but I can feel balanced
when I'm ready"

Side-of-the-eye point
"I still have these remaining unbalanced feelings"

Under-the-eye point
"I have my own reasons to feel unbalanced"

Under-the-nose point
"When I feel unbalanced, it makes me unhappy"

Under-the-mouth point
"I want to let my unbalanced feelings go"

Collarbone point
**"Having these unbalanced feelings caused me
to be stressed"**

Under-the-arm point
**"I accept I feel unbalanced, even if I still don't
understand the reasons"**

Top-of-the-head point
"I'm tired of being unbalanced"

Round 3 – Tap

Eyebrow point
"Finally I have to feel balanced"

Side-of-the-eye point
"I deserve to feel balanced and happy"

Under-the-eye point
"I am happy I can choose let my stress go"

Under-the-nose point
"I have the right to feel better and happier"

Under-the-mouth point
"I don't have to punish myself when I feel unbalanced"

Collarbone point
"It is important to me to feel balanced, so I can release anxiety and stress"

Under-the-arm point
"I choose not to feel unbalanced anymore"

Top-of-the-head point
"I will be very happy to feel balanced"

Confidence Builder - Develop Confidence from Within

The single best way to look confident is to simply be confident. Developing your inner confidence is a sure-fire way to look confident.

You can start by appreciating yourself a little more. Love yourself for who you are and what you are. You can put more emphasis on your strengths and accomplishments.

As for your weaknesses, find ways to correct them and transform them into strengths. Being on a constant state of improvement and self-appreciation is a great way to inspire confidence from within.

Script 5 - Love myself for who I am

Clearing of psychological reversal

Tap about 7 seconds for each statement on your karate point.

Continue tapping until you have finished saying all the following statements (Repeat psychological reversal three times):

- **Although I feel I don't love myself for who I am, I still love and fully accept that I have this bad feeling.**

- **Although I don't love myself for who I am for so long, I forgive myself for whatever I have done to contribute to the emotional pain.**

179

- Although I still feel I don't love myself for who I am
  and I have lots of good reasons for this feeling,
  I forgive the other people who have added to my bad feeling.

Tap (three rounds)

Eyebrow point
"I love myself for who I am"

Side-of-the-eye point
"I deserve to love myself every day"

Under-the-eye point
"I really deserve to love myself for who I am"

Under-the-nose point
"I have the right to love myself for who I am
and it makes me happy"

Under-the-mouth point
"I have the right to love myself for who I am
and it makes me happier"

Collarbone point
"People wish to love me for who I am"

Under-the-arm point
"I wish I could love myself forever"

Top-of-the-head point
"I will be very happy to love myself for who I am because I have every right"

Part 6 - <u>Bonus</u>
The Stress Release Tapping Challenge

This section is about EFT TAPPING and other strategies on how to overcome stress using natural and practical EFT.

Introduction

This section is about EFT TAPPING and other strategies on how to overcome stress, anxiety and panic attacks using natural and practical Tapping method.

Stress, anxiety, panic attacks and social anxiety are no simple matters as they can destroy lives and rob off freedom to live happily and normally.

However, coping with anxiety need not be complicated if only you know how to change yourself for the better, adapt a better lifestyle and habits and understand where your condition is coming from.

Do not be embarrassed with your condition because overcoming it is highly plausible. What is embarrassing is knowing what to do about it but choose not to act.

Managing your Stress

Stress can be caused by both real and imaginary situations. Often, these situations will make you feel threatened in some way and cause a certain stress response within your body. The way that the human body reacts to certain stressful situations can vary from one person to another.

However, the perceived threats and their resulting emotions can cause significant changes to the body's skin, systems, muscles, energy levels, and cells.

As luck would have it, there are numerous methods that you can use to cope with everyday stressors and help your body recover faster. However if you simply cannot find the time to engage in regular exercise, eat healthy, or achieve the recommended 8-10 hours of sleep, then practicing the Emotional Freedom Technique could be a better alternative that can help you manage your stress without consuming a lot of your time.

The EFT can help relieve a lot of your stress faster and more effectively than many other psychotherapeutic treatments can since it requires you to apply mediation, affirmation, and energy access techniques all at the same time.

It is also possible to perform EFT at your own leisure or to work with a licensed professional. Getting professional help is particularly recommended for individuals who are suffering from the loss of a loved one or those who have severe stress conditions such as PTSD which are caused by deep trauma.

Treating Anxiety

Although stress and anxiety are related concepts, anxiety generally involves a more prevalent sense of dread, fear, or apprehension. Nevertheless, certain levels of anxiety are also natural responses that can help you deal with certain stressful situations.

Brief levels of anxiety help to keep you alert by making your heart beat faster and your lungs pump harder. Such a heightened state of awareness makes you ready to jump to action at the slightest provocation.

In truth, anxiety only becomes a major issue when it changes from a brief period of alertness to a permanent state of fear. Chronic anxiety attacks can cause significant damage to your body and leave you at risk for several physical and mental health issues.

Although it can be difficult to permanently remove anxiety especially when it has become chronic, EFT can help you reduce the amount of anxiety that you feel on a daily basis.

The finger tapping technique helps you access the special energy meridians within your body and correct the bioelectrical short-circuiting caused by heightened levels of anxiety.

Using EFT to Reduce Anxiety

EFT makes use of the body's natural healing abilities to restore itself to its optimum condition. By doing away with more tedious and artificial treatment methods, you can recover at a much faster rate simply by harnessing the natural power of your own mind and body. As long as the technique is properly used, EFT can result in heightened feelings of happiness and even foster a sense of self-acceptance.

The application of the Emotional Freedom Technique is similar to the execution of traditional acupuncture methods. Participants are required to identify the exact locations of certain pressure points on the body's energy meridian lines and tap them in a specific progressive pattern. They must also simultaneously recite designated affirmations or scripts that address the specific problem that is causing them pain.

EFT affirmations need to be stated repeatedly in order to truly harness their full power. The scripts usually follow a certain structure, although many practitioners are still free to create their own variations.

One basic affirmation is, ***"Even though I have a/this (state your problem), I still wholeheartedly accept and love myself."***

1. Finding your Pressure Points

The body's energy system is composed of a set of interconnected meridian lines wherein your life energy is stored. The life energy is more commonly known as "ki" and can be accessed using the known pressure points underneath specific areas on your body.

Although no scientific study has yet been able to prove the existence of electromagnetic energy meridians within the human body, touching the specific pressure points on the body has been noted to cause feelings of relief and release.

Some of the well-known pressure points are commonly found on the face and on the upper extremities. The pressure points on the face include those along the brow bones, those beneath and on the outer corners of the eyes, those underneath the nose, and those on the chin.

There are also pressure points that can be found along the collar bones, on the wrists within your arms. The most accessible pressure points are those found on your fingertips. These points are also commonly used to trace and access other related points on the energy meridian.

Although it is possible for you to perform EFT on yourself, there is evidence suggesting that the technique becomes more effective if you allow another person to access your pressure points.

Having another person touch you puts you in a more heightened state of awareness since your brain will immediately register the sensation as a foreign intrusion.

Additionally, allowing another person to touch you will give you the opportunity to focus more on the feelings and affirmations that you wish to evoke in yourself.

It will be easier for you to link the sensations with the positive scripts and address the exact anxieties and stressors that you are currently experiencing.

Hopefully, your positive emotions and EFT experience will help you create a more positive association with the body parts that you only previously considered as sources of pain.

2. The Importance of Positive Affirmations

Although there is no proven link between the affirmations and the subsequent positive feelings, patients who are suffering from general anxiety or even those who are experiencing social anxiety will find that repeatedly stating and thinking of positive affirmations still generate significant results.

As long as you turn those positive affirmations into a habit, you will find that it becomes easier and easier for you to achieve your goals. After all, instead of thinking that something is impossible and giving up, you will be able to say, "I can do it!" instead and actually convince yourself that you can.

Likewise, you should always be on the lookout for the many negative scripts that you commonly encounter on a daily basis. You should learn to consciously replace such negative statements such as "I am not good enough", or "This is making me very anxious" into their positive counterparts.

By replacing anxiety with positivity, you will become more empowered and ready to face whatever situation or problem you may encounter along the way.

Useful EFT Affirmations

While the traditional EFT phrase is quite basic and easily adaptable, some practitioners could consider it far too general to be truly effective. For this reason, many practitioners would recommend that you create your own variations on the phrase so that you can specifically target your own personal ills and issues.

Those who are suffering from social anxieties such as public speaking can address the issue by saying, *"Even though I am afraid of speaking in front of large groups of people, I deeply love and accept myself."*

Meanwhile, those who have fears that are rooted in some type of childhood or past trauma can use the phrase, *"Even though I have this fear of snakes/dogs/cats/confined spaces/heights/darkness/my father's anger, I deeply love and accept myself."*

Finally, those who are suffering from more physical pain can use the phrase, *"Even though I have this stiff neck/pain on my lower back/throbbing on my left brow, I deeply love and accept myself."*

Creating Your Own Affirmations

By simply using the general format of first acknowledging your problem and finding self-acceptance despite these problems, it is possible for you to create affirmations that can address even your most specific issues.

As long as you are able to state just how much you love and accept yourself, you will be able to come up with a phrase that can help you get through any type of physical or emotional pain.

Some variations on the basic phrase are, *"I accept myself wholeheartedly even though I have _____."* *Another possible option is, "I love and deeply accept myself even though I have _____."*

3. EFT Steps

In order for the positive affirmations to be truly effective, you will have to consciously tune into the personal issues that you need to address. Anxieties are often caused by irrational fears, but they can also stem from long held feelings of loneliness, trauma, rejection, and depression.

Therefore, in order to successful remove those obstructions that are causing your pain, you will need to simultaneously think about the issue, tap on the specific pressure points and recite your affirmation of self-acceptance.

This way, you will be able to successfully replace the previous negative feeling, emotion, or pain with a more positive experience.

Almost immediately, you should be able to feel the positive energy flowing within your body. The pain and anxieties should also slowly begin to dissipate.

Continue tapping on your pressure points and reciting your affirmations until the feelings of pain and anxiety have completely disappeared.

Example

<u>Step 1 – Clearing of psychological reversal</u>

Tap about 5 seconds for each statement on your **karate point**. Continue tapping until you have finished saying all the following statements (Repeat psychological reversal 3 times):

- *Although I have fears about_____, I still love and fully accept myself.*

- *Although I don't always feel calm, I forgive myself for whatever I have done to contribute to the emotional pain.*

- *Although I fear of_____, I forgive the other people who have added to my fear.*

- *Although I have stress, I will forever love and fully accept myself.*

Step 2 – Tap

Here are the steps in tapping. There are three rounds. In each round repeat tapping about 5 seconds on each of the points. Start tapping your index and middle fingers on the following points of your body.

Here are the steps in tapping. Repeat tapping about 5 seconds on each of the points.

Start tapping your index and middle fingers on the following points of your body.

Tap **three** rounds:

Eyebrow point
"Fears about _____"

Side-of-the-eye point
"I can release my fears about _____"

Under-the-eye point
"Don't always feel calm"

Under-the-nose point
"Don't always feel good"

Under-the-mouth point
"Fear of _____"

Collarbone point
"I am reducing my fear of _____"

Under-the-arm point
"My stress causes me pain"

Top-of-the-head point
"My anxiety causes me emotional pain"

Nine Stress and Anxiety Management Strategies

Fact: Most cases of anxiety and panic attack happen outside the home away from family, especially at work, which is not surprising really because the workplace is a Mecca of stressors that elicit different negative emotions and thoughts – fear, insecurity and doubt.

Thus, learning how to effectively cope with anxiety and panic attacks while trying to maintain a normal life at work is vital in successfully overcoming your condition.

The purpose of this chapter is for you to learn how to adjust according to your condition and according to your environment. You have no total control over your job, responsibilities, challenges and problems, coworkers, superiors and clients, so the best way to cope effectively is still to adjust yourself.

To do these, you have to learn how to manage your condition and whatever factors you can control.

These nine anxiety management tips will walk you through a better life free of debilitating attacks. Although these are specifically designed to help sufferers at work, you will notice that these are actually practical approaches that anyone can apply in and out of the workplace.

All of these tips are all proven to relieve social anxiety and excessive worrying and help in managing other anxiety disorders and social phobias.

Live and breathe these coping mechanisms to successfully overcome anxiety and panic problems.

1 - *Know the boundaries*

It is a harsh reality, but the mere fact that you are able to maintain a job with anxiety problem (or disorder) is already something to be thankful about because most employers see your condition as a liability and hindrance to success – and it is for many people.

The first rule in coping with anxiety and panic attacks at work is to know the environment from all corners. That is the only way that you can conform to the demands of your work and be able to manage yourself while meeting those demands.

Stressors – things to be anxious about – will never disappear at work because they are part of every job. The sooner you accept that, the sooner you can adjust.

By doing so, you should be able to answer these questions:

- What are the demands and expectations of the employer?

- What are the limitations of your position and the limitation of your ability in fulfilling the responsibilities of that position?

- What are the tasks and who are the people you feel anxious to work with?

- How much work can you accept and decline without appearing incompetent?

- Who knows about your condition and how much of it is accepted by the employer?

By learning your job and the work environment on a full 360, you will also be able to identify your own anxiety and panic attack triggers at work.

The boundaries will be much clearer not only to you but to your coworkers as well. Your room to move around has to have four corners and four walls that when breached means red alert – a warning for you to step back a little, away from the afflicting effects of your condition.

Setting your own standards, guidelines and routines that conform to your boundaries is the ideal beginning of an effective management of anxiety and panic attacks.

You will be able to avoid whatever there is to be avoided and manage what is there to work at.

2 - Avoid triggers and alter what you cannot

Basically, things that give you extra pressure that you think you cannot handle are all potential triggers. The workplace is teeming with them.

Nonetheless, triggers are only harmful once you encounter them. Dormant triggers will cause you no trouble, reason why you have to know the boundaries to see where they are and how to avoid them.

Triggers are either avoidable or alterable. Avoid what you can and change what you cannot avoid.

How do you avoid them? Make set-ups and special arrangements if possible. Manage your time wisely so as not to coincide with some of them. Talk to people who have control over some conditions in your workplace like your superiors and coworkers. Take the initiative if need be because you will always be the first one to act on your condition.

If you fear speaking in public and there are other people in the team who can fill in, try talking to your boss and say that you might not be as effective in public speaking as you are in your desk work, not with your current condition, at least.

If you are not comfortable doing a specific task, ask if you can do something else to work on your strength and be a bigger help in the process. If you are often given with a lot of tasks more than what you can properly manage, learn to say no.

If somebody in the team can help you, learn to delegate. If you find a certain co-employee hard to deal with, avoid talking or having a confrontation with that person when not needed to begin with.

How about if you cannot avoid them? Learn how to alter. Some things are just a matter of proper management.

You do not have to panic on a deadline if you can master time management and discipline.

If panic attack often troubles you as tasks start to swarm in, perhaps, it is best to go to work earlier than usual just to have a leeway for extra tasks.

If you fear being reprimanded because of your late time-in, learn to wake-up earlier and move faster.

Screen what you can screen and accept that some things are meant to add to your ordeal. Learn where your weaknesses lie.

3- Accept your symptoms

Many anxiety and panic attack sufferers are embarrassed of their symptoms, which even add to their worries. However, symptoms are symptoms and unless you accept them as they are, you would not be able to understand them fully and manage them properly.

Aside from the fearful thoughts, exaggerated and illogical worries, upsetting emotions and breaking of spirit, physical symptoms also accompany anxiety and panic attacks and these symptoms are more embarrassing than the actual conditions for many sufferers.

Manifestations as shaking, heavy sweating, freezing, nausea, hyperventilation and chest pain are hard to hide (sufferers always fear of being embarrassed because of these symptoms), but the thing is, you need support from your coworkers to help you out during such time of emergency.

Thus, accepting, identifying and sharing your most prominent symptoms are a must.

People around you cannot accept who you are if you yourself do not accept what you are suffering from.

Sharing your condition with your trusted coworkers is most especially essential in coping with your condition successfully if your symptoms already interfere with your daily activities, affecting performance and professionalism.

Imagine the horror of your coworkers when you suddenly have erratic breathing due to a deluge of paperwork with strict deadlines without them having any idea why it is happening.

Hiding some symptoms is still possible if you are not really comfortable sharing it with others. However, remind yourself that not all symptoms pass by without apparent effects in your performance and status.

4 - Take a break

Being workaholic is admirable, but it is still borderline abuse of body, not a good thing to do if you suffer from panic attack and anxiety problems. Stress buildup is one of the most common causes of sudden anxiety and panic attacks.

Curtailing that buildup will provide you more free space to absorb new ones to come.

Relaxing your mind and body from time to time before they give in to stress, pressure and fear will allow your body to neutralize hormonal changes that cause mental and emotional instability.

It can be as simple as taking deep breaths in the midst of a heated meeting, or 20 seconds of silence and blankness by closing your eyes and practicing mindfulness meditation.

If you've been staring on piles of papers and computer monitors for hours, crunching numbers and analyzing data, calm your senses by focusing your eyes on distant objects and looking into cool colors (e.g. green and blue).

Drinking water (or any beverages from the listed "anti-anxiety" foods in this book) every 30 minutes to one hour will also replenish your energy and relax your dehydrating muscles. Skip the coffee break and instead, take short naps or at least, time to close your eyes and temporarily shut down your brain from over-thinking.

Walking and stretching for a minute have also been seen to improve chances of warding off anxiety and panic attack by stabilizing blood circulation and blood pressure.

5 - *Be conscious of your breathing*

Hyperventilation is usually the first sign of an impending panic attack. It starts to take toll on your body even before your mind notices it.

According to experts, stopping hyperventilation, which is essentially the first stage of an attack, is usually sufficient in stopping the attack altogether.

Normalizing the breathing pattern already lowers blood pressure, restores healthy blood flow, calms muscles and clears your mind. A simple hyperventilating remedy can definitely take you a long way.

As you have been told to understand, identify and accept your symptoms, you should be aware of the changes in your mood, way of thinking and physiological functions to clearly determine when and how to act.

When your breathing already starts to get shallow and rapid with irregular interval, all you have to do is to slow down by practicing recommended breathing techniques.

The best breathing exercise is the 5-2-5 diaphragmatic breathing. In this technique, you are to inhale using your stomach and not your chest. Inhale slowly for five seconds and feel your stomach expand, protruding to its maximum capacity and holding that air for two seconds. Then, exhale slowly again for five seconds. Repeat this breathing exercise until you feel your heart rate slow down.

Humming while exhaling also brings a different kind of relaxation, which is usually practiced under Bhramari Pranayam, a type of meditative yoga that incorporates breathing exercise and physical relaxation.

While in a relaxed position, close your eyes and focus your mind on your breathing and not on any distractions. Plug your ears with your index fingers, then let the air out of your chest slowly while vibrating your throat with a humming sound.

Experts consider this kind of breathing exercise a form of self-hypnosis and meditation combined.

It might be hard at first, but understand that the only best way to counteract palpitation is by reversing the speed meter, going south in as much controlled fashion as possible.

Forget the paper bag technique, which is perhaps the most popular short-term relief for acute panic attacks. That is so 90s.

The paper bag technique is a breathing exercise that lets a patient breathe in and out through a close-ended paper bag to circulate carbon dioxide back for inhalation.

Carbon dioxide is said to reduce symptoms of anxiety and panic attacks.

Many medical experts no longer recommend this traditional relief as there are evidences indicating possible worsening of panicking due to the sudden increase of carbon dioxide in the bloodstream.

On the other hand, the decrease of oxygen supply to the brain makes it harder for a patient to calm down and focus.

6 - Use positive affirmations

Who would pat your back first but you?

A person who has high anxiety and is in the brink of having anxiety attack has already activated his automated negative self-talking side – the part of his brain that decides for the future, concludes for other people and accepts things based on pessimistic predisposition rather than logical reasoning, all for the worse.

Fear-based thoughts start to creep in as signs and symptoms of anxiety begin. Suppress those thoughts that educe negative emotions by countering them with positive affirmations.

Affirmations are motivating statements, mantras that reassure your ability and worth.

The purpose of affirmations is to strengthen your resolve and sense of self-appreciation – to make yourself believe in the best possibilities and not on the worst case scenarios in your head.

You might think *"I can't do this because I might have an anxiety attack"* when faced with a tough task at work. Counter this by saying *"I am far stronger than my anxiety problem."*

Whenever you feel weak and fragile because of your condition, talk to yourself and say *"It takes more than this to bring me down"* or *"Anxiety won't kill me because I am tough."*

You have to believe every single word you say to convince yourself and live up to your own expectations.

Every time you feel down, afraid, doubtful and unworthy, find reasons why you are better than those.

Repeat affirmations to yourself all over and over again – before you go to work, as you enter the office, before talking with your boss, before going to a presentation and while leaving for home.

Close the day with a powerful mantra, like *"I did great today; I'll definitely do better tomorrow."*

7- *Set your goal and look forward to achieving it*

You need to find a strong reason to strive harder at work because it will be pointless to try to overcome anxiety and panic attacks for nothing.

Do it for yourself, for your family, for your dreams, for the most-hankered position you always wanted, for a salary raise or for fame. Know what you want and have a strong connection to that.

Visualization is an effective way of inculcating your goals in your mind, clear enough to fight fears and insecurities intrinsically.

This is called mindfulness technique or mind-body meditation. Everyone can easily practice this when fear and apprehension start to set in.

Take a relaxing position, preferably sitting straight while comfortably leaning on your back. Your shoulders and head should be relaxed. Close your eyes while doing deep, slow breathing.

Focus all your attention on your breathing – no worries, no distractions. Do not entertain whatever discomfort and pain you have, as much as you can.

Now, visualize your dreams coming into reality, as detailed as possible. If you aspire to be the boss in your company, picture yourself sitting in a high-back executive chair in your own office with your subordinates.

If you dream of becoming a millionaire, picture yourself sipping red wine on top of a yacht while sailing across the Mediterranean Sea. Perhaps, visualize the house you want to live in when you get rich, complete with a full-lap pool and rooftop Jacuzzi.

As you see your goals coming into life, use affirmations and tell yourself that you can do it, you can achieve them and that you will succeed because you are good and you deserve it.

This will strengthen your resolve and raise your spirit into accomplishing the impossible, even if it means fighting despite fear and doubts.

The sources of your anxiety and panic attacks are all in your head. It is but proper to try to solve your weaknesses first starting with the power of your mind.

8 - Set realistic standards and expectations

Panic attack happens when you fail to meet your own or somebody else's expectations, whether as results of your own actions or as results of your wishful thinking, like in the case of expecting the outcomes of events.

Hence, lowering your own standards and expectations to a realistic level will also lower your chances of not hitting the very high mark you originally set.

Aspiring for the better is ideal to achieve higher success and bring out the best in you. However, if "better" is essentially unattainable at a given time, the result just becomes "worse."

Consequentially, you panic for not delivering as you expect it to be, thinking that your expectations are all the same for everyone. What you do not know is that most high expectations are all in your head.

Most sufferers of anxiety and panic attacks set ideal standards and expectations that are not necessarily attainable given their current ability and situation.

For instance, they intend to impress their boss to have a salary raise or promotion but do not necessarily back up that standard with ability and knowledge. In the end, they fail but only by their own standards, embracing their own expectations as the general expectations of all the people around them.

Come to think of it. If they completely fail in their jobs, they wouldn't be staying any longer, would they?

Hope for the best but prepare for the worse, or as the saying goes. *Hope* is the word, not expect.

Best case scenarios are ideal but are not always bound to happen, so do not be disappointed and lose hope when they fail.

Or rather, do not panic because not meeting your expectations is not the end of the world or your own career.

Standards are just delineations so you can see how high you can go, provided that all the odds are on your side (life is a bet, so don't expect too much).

9 - *Get professional help*

When things get out of hand and cannot seem to be controlled anymore, the time has probably come to leave matters to the hands of professionals.

Clinical psychologists, psychotherapists, psychiatrists, clinicians and licensed mental health experts all specialize in diagnosing mental disorders and treating them to avoid worsening.

At some point, there might be a need to consult them rather than do self-diagnosis and self-treatment.

Unusual rush of negative thoughts and emotions with palpable manifestations in the form of symptoms clearly means there is anxiety and panic problems. The onset of these mental and emotional changes with the sudden strike of fear means an attack is starting to happen.

Experiencing attacks very often might mean the development of anxiety and panic disorders.

However, unlike an attack that you can simply distinguish from normal worrying, a disorder needs proper diagnosis using widely recognized medical testing and procedures. Formal diagnosis is also required to have medications and clinical treatments.

Moreover, many companies acknowledge the special attention for such conditions of their employees only with proper diagnosis and treatment.

If you want to request for some adjustments and special set-up for your case, you might have to present formal documents that your condition really exists. Likewise, there are employers who accept employees with anxiety and panic disorders for limited roles in the business only with the concurrence of treatments.

A business that is already going south seeks the help of consultants to bounce back. The same goes with anxiety and panic disorder sufferers.

Remember that your job is your livelihood. It is just proper to safeguard it and do everything to fix what is there to be fixed.

Do not be embarrassed about your situation because you and your family's future depends on it.

8. Following Practical Ways to Overcoming Stress and Anxiety

Battling the symptoms of anxiety and panic attacks is not an easy task because you have your own mind as your enemy. In the previous chapter, you have learnt ways to effectively overcome attacks at work and prevent them.

But before that, you have to master the management of your condition first through healthy habits and proper lifestyle changes.

Autogenic training

This technique is a self-performed psychotherapy where you practically program your mind into believing in your own abilities to achieve your dreams and goals.

For 15 minutes before you start your day every day, have a moment of stillness and silence complemented by a breathing exercise, inhaling and exhaling slowly as you clear your mind of any distractions.

For the whole duration of this exercise, think of only happy thoughts and mental images that inspire and motivate you.

Doing this exercise everyday will program your mind to memorize the sense and feeling of happiness, free of stress and worries and make it a part of your natural fight-or-flight response.

As the term implies, it prompts your mind to automatically adapt to stress and anxiety by adjusting itself to the peaceful setting that you use every single day.

Psychotherapists believe that autogenic training purges your autonomic nervous system of harmful mindsets.

Sleeping for seven to eight hours a day

How basic can it get with sleeping?
Unfortunately, this is a very common culprit in anxiety attacks that many sufferers least suspect.

It has been proven in studies over and over again that the lack of mental rest significantly lowers mental agility and clarity, making it hard to focus and reason out logically during times of pressure.

Illogical fear and excessive worrying usually set in when the mind has no enough capacity to screen thoughts because of insufficient replenishment and revitalization.

Sleep is so powerful that it can permanently delete illogical thoughts that you've created during the past day, retaining only those that are mostly usable and factual. As a matter of fact, simply taking a nap for 15 minutes can already boost your mental agility by 20%.

Sleeping for at least seven hours also increases dopamine and melatonin levels in the body, two hormones that are responsible in maintaining sense of pleasure and happiness.

Talk and have physical contact with someone

In a study, researchers observed that people who often talk with happy friends also have higher levels of dopamine in the body, a feel-good and pleasure hormone that counters the secretion of stress hormones, which are directly responsible for the surge of negative emotions and accompanying manifestations (in the form of symptoms).

An idle mind is the devil's playground and for someone who suffers from anxiety and panic problems, that is very much true.

Stimulate your mind with fun activities that will take away your focus from negative thoughts.

Prevent panic and anxiety attacks with anti-anxiety foods

You are what you eat – your health, mood, behavior and what else, appearance! Nutrients and chemicals play starring roles when it comes to beating anxiety, panic disorders and social anxiety because they have direct impact on your emotions and thoughts as they control the secretion of hormones and chemicals that stir your brain.

Foods manifest as emotions because they are responsible for your mental and physical health. Different emotions and way of thinking can be improved if only you have the right ingredients to produce positive emotions.

There is a growing interest in the international medical community in the prevention and maintenance of mental disorders using diets and nutrition. Rather than discovering treatments, many scientists now look into the role of chemicals and lifestyle in the development of diseases.

The foods listed in this guide are a result of years of intense research directed towards the treatment and management of anxiety and panic disorders. These foods are highly recommended by therapists and nutritionists to beat and manage anxiety attacks, panic attacks and social anxiety more effectively.

9. "Anti-Anxiety" And "Anti-Panic Attack" Foods

First, here are 18 "anti-anxiety" and "anti-panic attack" foods that should be available in your refrigerator. You might be surprised that these simple foods can bring very complex benefits and actions to your condition.

1. Dark chocolate

Care to know why broken-hearted individuals love indulging on chocolates to uplift their moods? Well, it is actually a matter of choice, but probably subconscious at that.

A study conducted at the University of California-San Diego's School of Medicine proved that people who show increasing depressive symptoms tend to eat chocolate more to appease their emotions and help them feel better. It is like a subconscious craving where the mind tells you that you need it to become mentally and emotionally stable.

For a person who has mental disturbance due to anxiety and panic attacks, it is important to regain composure and control by lowering negative emotions and thoughts. Chocolates will help with that. As a great source of flavonoid, it will also make it easier for you to relax, both mentally and physically.

Dark chocolates, in particular, are especially helpful because their flavonol and polyphenol contents can lower blood pressure, one thing that people on the brink of anxiety and panic attacks badly need. The calming effect is almost instantaneous.

Because chocolate also triggers the production of the relaxing and pain-relieving hormone called endorphin, eating a single bar might already help you alleviate the mild physical symptoms in minutes.

Consider dark chocolate as your non-drug medicine.

On prior studies, dark chocolate is also proven to contain high amounts of phenyl ethylamine, a compound that triggers the brain to produce a chemical that mimics happiness and calmness called anandamide.

In a way, dark chocolate can work as a natural sedative. Eating a bar of it can already lower your production of cortisol, a stress hormone that triggers the manifestation of symptoms of Generalized Anxiety Disorder (GAD) and Social Anxiety Disorder.

Just watch your portions carefully...and do count the calories (although dark chocolates obviously have lower or no sugar at all). You do not want to solve your anxiety and panic disorders just to give birth to depression due to becoming overweight.

2. Avocado

Many people love making a facial mask out of it rather than eating it because of its high fat content (four times more than a finger of banana), but do you know that avocado is effective in delaying the aggravation of anxiety and panic disorders, as well as phobias?

Avocado has the richest amount of glutathione among all fruits. This substance is essential in the nourishment of the liver and in the reduction of fat absorption, which when left uncontrolled can contribute to increased oxidative damage of the brain (Yes! Despite having "higher" amount of fat itself).

Oxidative damage is said to be one of the reasons why phobia starts to develop starting from the brain itself (the same with dementia, Alzheimer's disease and age-related memory decline).

A piece of avocado a day already offers you generous amounts of lutein, folate, vitamin E and beta-carotene, nutrients that aid in regulating the brain's healthy function.

3. Cashew

Do you know that scientists have linked zinc deficiency to the development of depression and anxiety disorder?

If you are suffering from anxiety and panic attacks, there is a big chance that you do not get your recommended dietary allowance (RDA) of zinc every day.

Unfortunately, even multivitamins seldom contain 100% of your zinc needs (since it is a mineral that is less concentrated on by dietary supplement manufacturers). The solution – an ounce of cashew!

A single ounce of cashew can already provide you 11% of your RDA. Because humans have no way of storing zinc in their bodies, it is a must to replenish your supply every single day.

Chop it, toast it, crush it, bake it – you name it! This is a very versatile food, so you will have 101 ways of eating it towards a better mental health.

4. Garlic

Do not underestimate the power of garlic in treating your anxiety problem from within. This bulb is rich in allicin, a compound with antimicrobial property that is also seen to be potent against heart diseases, carcinomas and flu.

More than anything else, though, allicin can alleviate symptoms of stress and anxiety while also providing you a good supply of antioxidant to fight cell damages and premature ageing.

Garlic will help you tremendously in preventing the aggravation of simpler anxiety and panic attacks into more serious anxiety and panic disorders.

In any case, garlic's natural ability to directly enhance the immune system will help you fight the physical symptoms of anxiety, which include muscle spasms, body pains, headaches, heavy sweating and digestive problem, among others.

5. Oyster

Going back to zinc, oysters are heavyweights when it comes to zinc content. Half a dozen (which is the average serving size in restaurants) of this scrumptious shellfish already contains more than half of your daily needs of zinc, not bad in managing anxiety problems.

Experts believe that oyster's natural property that makes it a globally-renowned aphrodisiac is also beneficial to anxiety and panic disorder sufferers.

By increasing your serotonin production (perhaps with indirect effect to libido), you stabilize your mood and emotions, which can help you avoid anxiety and panic attacks on a daily basis in the first place.

It is better if you will eat the oyster as fresh as possible, preferably with less cooking involved to preserve its nutrients and contained compounds (remember that oysters tend to be overcooked with multiple baking, searing and boiling).

6. *Walnut*

There is no solid direct link between walnut and anxiety and panic attacks, but scientists see a really promising benefit of this crunchy nut to people who often experience such attacks.

A study at the Tufts University looked into its benefits to brain ageing, and the results are more than satisfying. What's surprising, though, is one of its recorded benefits to the brain is a possible support for cognitive health as well.

Researchers found out that eating walnuts a day is highly supportive of brain function that can prevent, if not delay, the onset of mental disorders, anxiety and panic disorders included.

You are also guaranteed to get a decent supply of polyphenol, omega-3 fatty acid and alpha-linoleic acid that are all seen to preserve memory.

Walnut has been seen to effectively counterbalance adrenaline in the body (that makes panicking even more harmful), as well as lower blood pressure in people who are already experiencing the attack.

Putting a small pack of fresh or toasted walnut in your bag wherever you go is a smart way to alleviate signs when you already feel like having an anxiety and panic attack.

7. Oatmeal

This is the ultimate comfort food for people suffering from anxiety and panic attacks, both young and old. Why is it a must-include in your diet?

First, there is a study concluding that children who eat oatmeal for breakfast have lower chances of throwing tantrums during the day, have higher energy and mental alertness, have sharper memory and are more emotionally stable than those who do not eat breakfast at all.

This is the reason why oatmeal is highly recommended for children with separation anxiety.

Second, a bowl of oatmeal has an amount of soluble fiber that is more than what you will need for the day. Called beta-glucan, it will make you feel fuller every time you eat and at the same time, will decrease your fat absorption that again, can contribute to the reduction of oxidative damage to your brain.

Third, oatmeal triggers your brain to secrete more serotonin, which is also called the feel-good hormone.

Needless to say, a person suffering from anxiety and panic attacks has very low amount of this hormone, disabling him/her from staying calm and making it harder for a person to stay mentally focused.

A good dose of serotonin is one of the best ways to fight anxiety naturally.

Lastly, oatmeal provides the magnesium that you need, a mineral that when at low amounts in the body can lead to anxiety, depression, higher stress level, memory decline and irritability.

Magnesium has direct impact on your mental and emotional state, so you should better take it seriously.

8. Saltwater fatty fishes

Salmon, tuna, mackerel, sardine and trout are highly recommended for anxiety and panic attack sufferers because of their rich amounts of omega-3 fatty acid and vitamin B complex.

Dozens of scientific studies have already confirmed the benefits of this fatty acid against mental degradation, which makes a person more prone to the development of mental disorders.

Omega-3 fatty acid enhances mental function by increasing the amount of oxygen supplied to the brain. At the same time, higher oxygen level in the blood also means stronger respiratory system.

This will help you prepare in fighting anxiety and panic attacks since many of their symptoms directly affect your breathing, blood circulation and pressure and organ function.

Because anxiety and panic disorders are two of the most common mental disorders among people, adding a serving of saltwater fatty fish in your meal everyday will already pull you miles away from experiencing an attack anytime soon.

Salmon in particular, can nudge your brain into producing more serotonin, which you will definitely need in controlling your condition towards living a normal life.

Based on a study conducted by the health center Kaiser Permanente in California, salmon can also lower your mood of hostility by 20%! Your family and friends will surely love it (especially if you often throw your anger at them during attacks).

9. Sunflower seed

If you are looking for a beneficial snack for your condition, you will definitely never go wrong with sunflower seed. Forget popcorn and chips for now because sunflower might just save you from pain and embarrassment during an anxiety or panic attack.

Sunflower seed is an excellent source of folate and magnesium. These nutrients are what your body needs to produce its sufficient supply of dopamine, a type of neurotransmitter that has direct responsibility over the emulation of "pleasure."

This particular neurotransmitter helps a lot in the alleviation of anxiety symptoms that might lead to anxiety attack (and subsequently, anxiety disorder).

Nibbling a sunflower seed will help you relax by allowing you to focus your attention on something else rather than entertain your negative thoughts and emotions.

As you eat it, its nutrients will then find their way to your system, allowing you to fight anxiety and panic attacks in both practical and scientific ways.

10. Almond

There are clinical observations that indicate how effective munching, chewing and nibbling can be as simple yet effective reliefs for anxiety.

Some researchers say that the act of "eating" whets the appetite which is considered a positive emotion (usually partnered with excitement, joy and fulfillment).

This is the reason why "medical" chewing gums are marketed as reliefs for addiction, anxiety and panic attacks.

When it comes to crunch, almond will definitely win. It is a snack full of "anti-anxiety" nutrients that can help you toughen your defense against attacks and other symptoms.

It is a good source of zinc, magnesium, cyanacobalamin and vitamin E that can keep you healthy in the inside and the outside.

11. *Banana*

This fruit is a standout because it is a great source of potassium. However, not many people know that banana is also one of the very few fruits and grains that naturally contain melatonin, a hormone that in humans regulates sleep patterns and enables deep relaxation.

Eating a finger of banana before trying to get to sleep after an anxiety or panic attack will help you restore your energy and mental clarity with deep relaxation.

Melatonin also regulates physiological functions in humans such as blood pressure and heart rate, so it will be easier for you to relax when agitated during an attack.

This is also recommended to those who cannot go to sleep because of the symptoms of anxiety.

Making banana a regular part of your meal will help you stay calm for the whole day.

12. Orange

If there is one fruit that therapists recommend you bring anywhere if you have an anxiety or panic disorder, it would be orange.

Its tough skin makes it highly portable while its vitamin C content is a great way to counteract the implications of too much stress and anxiety in your body.

According to Dr. Pam Peeke of the University of Maryland, orange is a very effective replacement to gums and cigarette when you are feeling nervous.

Many people get fixated orally when nervous, while some tinker and fiddle restlessly. A piece of orange will solve all of that.

13. *Green leafy vegetables*

What do spinach, broccoli, arugula and Swiss chard have in common?

They are all green leafy vegetables, and they are rich in vitamin B complex – thiamine, riboflavin, niacin, pantothenic acid, pyridoxine and cobalamin.

How can they help you in overcoming and managing anxiety and panic attacks successfully?

That is by boosting the production of your three feel-good hormones: dopamine, serotonin and norepinephrine.

Eating green leafy vegetables everyday will lower your chances of having anxiety and panic attacks in the first place because you are secured with higher levels of counteracting hormones. They work like maintenance drugs, only filled with more antioxidants and other vitamins.

Besides, according to a research released in the peer-review journal, *Journal of Neuroscience Nursing*, irritability, nervousness and depression are all related to lower levels of pyridoxine (vitamin B6) in the body.

Avoid getting nervous easily by getting your fill of green leafy vegetables daily.

14. Milk

Aside from the fact that milk is very good for your bones and teeth, this all-time favorite beverage is also helpful for coping with anxiety and panic disorders because of its whey protein content.

This specific type of protein enhances tryptophan level in the body, a kind of amino acid that is considered an essential building block of the feel-good hormone serotonin.

According to a study made in Denmark, simply drinking a glass of milk everyday already boosts your serotonin level by up to 43%. This is more than what you need to stay away from anxiety and panic attacks for the entire day.

Also, drinking milk is very relaxing for many people, probably because it is associated with childhood when problems are still way ahead.

15. Cheese bread or cheese cake

What makes this dessert special? It is packed with carbohydrates for physical energy and protein for mental alertness, exactly what you need to ward off aggravation of physical symptoms of anxiety.

Being anxious consumes huge amount of energy that is why worrying alone is already physically and mentally draining.

If you have to go with sweets, go with cheese bread or cheese cake instead.

16. Asparagus

Asparagus has negative calories, meaning you will consume more calories in chewing it than what you can actually take from eating it.

This makes asparagus the perfect "binge snack" for mood eaters – people who experience increased appetite when sad, nervous, afraid and agitated (you also probably tend to binge uncontrollably when under stress). Go nibble all you want; you won't get fat.

Most importantly, asparagus is rich in folate that boosts your dopamine level (a pleasure hormone). It will aid you in keeping your cool when fidgeting starts to set in.

If you are not into green snacks, try broiled-crisp asparagus. It tastes like junk food with the nutrients you'll expect from a super food.

17. Berries

Speaking of super food, berries are some of the most nutritious foods in the planet, directly putting them on top of nutrition ladders of all standards. Their antioxidant and vitamin levels are crazy – just way over the top.

Raspberry, blackberries, wolfberry, blueberry, acai berry and even strawberry all contain polyphenols that regulate blood pressure, making you stronger against the symptoms of anxiety and panic attacks such as erratic heart rate, heavy sweating and breathing problem.

At the same time, their antioxidants will protect your brain cells from acquiring oxidative damages and undergoing premature cell death, delaying, if not preventing, the development of mental disorders in effect, including anxiety and panic disorders.

More recent studies also link ketone, an organic compound mostly present in berries (especially in raspberries), to the improved regulation of serotonin in the body.

Experts also suggest the use of this compound as an appetite-suppressant because it effectively suppresses binge eating that occurs on mood eaters.

One German study that involved 120 individuals measured the level of anxiety and stress on those who took berries rich in vitamin C and those who did not take anything prior to the test.

All of them were subjected to public speaking, which clearly separated those with social anxiety.

By the end of the test, those who took berries had lower blood pressures and stress hormones in their body, clearly resolving that berries can help alleviate the symptoms of social anxiety and fear of the public.

18. Chamomile Tea

Chamomile is the ultimate tea for anxiety sufferers – a must-try for those who already developed more harmful disorders. It is calming, relaxing and soothing. But why is it the king of anxiety-relieving teas?

First, it significantly alleviates symptoms of Generalized Anxiety Disorder (GAD). In a clinical study by the University of Pennsylvania to gauge its effectiveness against GAD, 57 patients were administered with chamomile in the form of supplement for two months.

After the testing period, all patients reported impressive and satisfactory results, finally putting chamomile on top of the "anti-anxiety" foods.

Although supplement was used instead of tea in this test, there are evidences that the same benefits are to be expected for both forms.

Second, the University of Maryland Medical Center found out that chamomile tea relaxes nerves and stimulates the brain into producing more sleep hormones despite mental agitation and physical distress.

If you are having a hard time sleeping because of anxiety, sipping a cup of chamomile tea before hitting the sack is very likely to give you deep slumber.

This tea has an instant effect, so this is absolutely a perfect substitution for coffee and other beverages.

You can buy readily prepared tea bags, but if you have chamomile in your backyard, you can make your own tea by steeping three tablespoonful of powdered dried flower for 10 minutes.

10. Avoiding Common Anxiety Trigger Foods

After learning the importance of diet in the management of anxiety and panic problems and identifying the foods that work best for your condition, the next step is to avoid those that contribute to the aggravation of your condition.

Discipline is important to successfully overcome panic and anxiety attacks. Like in any disease, there is a diet regimen that you should strictly follow to keep your cool and be less sensitive to triggers.

By avoiding these five common anxiety-trigger foods, you will also lower your chances of experiencing panic and anxiety attacks.

1. Coffee

You know coffee is bad for someone who has anxiety and panic disorder, but somehow, giving up a hot brew completely is not as simple as it seems.

This is because coffee has an addicting chemical that makes you want it more all the time. However, if you are damn serious about overcoming your condition, you will need to give up coffee without a second thought.

The caffeine in coffee stimulates the central nervous system. It has been observed in studies that the same amount of coffee given to those with anxiety and panic disorders create and worsen symptoms, but do not elicit the same effects from those without the disorders.

Unfortunately, decaf does not help much because in tests, caffeinated and decaffeinated coffees both triggered the same symptoms at almost the same rate (although experts imply that high-quality decaffeinated coffees according to brand and manufacturer might make a small difference).

2. Soda

Like coffee, soda has caffeine and worse, the diet versions also have aspartame, a sugar replacement that is also linked to irritability, agitation, mood swings and to some extent, depression. Caffeine and aspartame are also both headache triggers, making soda even more dangerous to those who show headache and nausea as their symptoms.

3. Alcohol

Alcohol badly affects behavior and emotion even for people without any mental disorder.

How much damage can it do for those who are battling anxiety and panic attacks?

Alcohol exaggerates everything in your head – fear, sadness, insecurity, depression. Although it does provide temporary calmness and relaxation, it can still be the opposite when abused.

Unfortunately for alcohol, the limitation marker is not as visible as it should be.

For people with advanced anxiety disorder, the increased lactic acid and sugar in the blood can lead to aggravated irritation and extended panic attacks, taking away their ability to sleep according to their biological clocks and truly relax when rested.

4. Monosodium Glutamate (MSG)

MSG is not the food in itself, but you will be surprised to learn how much MSG you are taking every year. It is available everywhere – in your chips, Asian cuisines, fast-food fries and burgers, soups, frozen meats and a lot more.

Currently, there is little evidence that MSG does trigger panic attacks. However, records of clinical observations are enough to prod experts into finding the link with more studies.

Until facts are established, it is advisable that you stay away from this artificial flavor enhancer for now. It may not trigger panic attack in you, but it will surely trigger migraine.

Other flavor enhancers to watch out for are autolyzed yeast, kombu extract and sodium caseinate.

5. Deli meats

Who doesn't love sausages?

Deli meats in general are full of additives and preservatives, chemicals that are proven to aggravate anxiety and lower ability to relax. Sulfites and nitrites, in particular, might trigger panic attack by altering healthy hormone secretion.

In children, deli meats are said to worsen Attention Deficit Hyperactivity Disorder (ADHD) and Attention Deficit Disorder (ADD) as they lower a person's ability to concentrate and clear his/her mind from the rush of negative thoughts and emotions.

Conclusion

I hope this book was able to help you really master the Tapping Therapy Technique and it makes you such a huge difference in the lives of those you touch, yourself as well as others, I'm sure!

I hope this book was able to help you really to be able to realize the positive and significant benefits EFT can give you especially when combined with the principles and laws of attraction.

Now you can gain the many advantages of feeling prosperous and attracting money and financial abundance into your life and letting go of all the negative things that hinder or limit you from achieving the things that you really desire and at the same time change the way you feel about so many things and influence your attitude and beliefs towards money in just a short time (5 minutes at least).

Now you can tap on some meridian points even without the help of a professional therapist as this eBook comes with handy EFT tapping scripts which you can utilize and share with your loved ones to help them change the way they view money and attract financial abundance as well.

I hope this book was able to help you open your mind to the healing possibilities of EFT. In the first chapter, we have revisited what EFT is and how it can heal you in the process. The succeeding chapters briefly discussed the primary aspects of weight loss such as the connection of food and emotions as well as how a person's perspective of themselves impacts their success.

Now you can TAKE ACTION. In the book, applications of EFT to curb cravings, increase metabolism and increase self-acceptance have been discussed. Simple EFT exercises were included to help you start your healing.

The next step is to practice putting the skills you have learned into action. You will improve your life and you will certainly attract money and financial abundance into your life. Practice The Tapping Therapy every day for 5 minutes, that's all!

Finally, if you enjoyed this book, please take the time to share your thoughts and post a review on Amazon. It'd be greatly appreciated!

Thank you and good luck!

Ben Buckland

Printed in Great Britain
by Amazon